Exploring the Environmental Upsides of COVID-19 Lockdowns

Sana

Table of Contents

Chapter 1: Introduction

1.1   Background and Context

In December 2019, a novel coronavirus called 2019-nCoV (better known now as SARS-CoV-2) was discovered in Wuhan, China after several individuals fell ill with pneumonia (Zhu et al., 2020). This virus is responsible for causing the disease COVID-19, which is a flu-like illness associated with a fever, pneumonia, and numerous other symptoms. (Stawicki et al., 2020). As a response, measures were taken to limit social interaction and the movement of people to prevent the transmission of the disease. Highly contagious, SARS-CoV-2 spread around the globe until COVID-19 reached every continent aside from Antarctica, which led to its classification as a pandemic (Berlinger, 2020; World Health Organization [WHO], 2020b). As of April 16th, 2021, there have been over 139 million cases worldwide and more than 2.9 million deaths (Johns Hopkins Center for Systems Science and Engineering [JHU CSSE], 2021). Since the novel coronavirus has proliferated around the world, social distancing and lockdown measures such as school closures, travel bans, and quarantine have been imposed in various countries (Dunford et al., 2020; Salcedo et al., 2020). As a result, an estimated 4.4 billion people around the world have experienced some sort of lockdown (Bates et al., 2020). This has led to a global "natural experiment," whereby a major intervention outside of human control is providing an opportunity to study its effects on different aspects of society (Thomson, 2020).

1.2   Problem Statement and Research Question

The unprecedented lockdown and continued social distancing measures have led to a multitude of global effects, including a large decline in travel and economic activity that has led to documented impacts on the natural environment. However, the effects that a human health crisis and its subsequent medical and public health responses can have on the environment are not well understood because research in the field of environmental health has historically focused on observing effects in the opposite direction: That is, research has focused on identifying the impacts of environmental risks on human health. This is understandable given the serious threat that the climate crisis and increasing environmental degradation pose to our planet and our society.

Environmental changes are leading to inherent impacts on public health, which have been discussed and documented extensively. One crucial finding is the negative impact of pollution (such as air and lead pollution) on human health, with effects disproportionately impacting children and lower-income and marginalized communities (Dockery et al., 1993; Landrigan et al., 2017; Needleman et al., 1979; Ransom & Pope, 1992). In addition, there is evidence of the effects of climate change on human health, such as increased morbidity and mortality from extreme heat (Patz et al., 2005). Though anthropogenic climate change is a process that is currently unfolding, public health consequences are already being observed. Workshops and panels have critically explored this relationship, with scholars siting the need for an integrated approach to understanding environmental impacts on public health in order to prepare for a sustainable, healthy future (Institute of Medicine, 2001; Institute of Medicine, 2013). In addition, international agencies such as the World Health Organization (WHO) have published reports that classify global impacts stemming from these environmental risks and analyze the implications of these findings (Prüss-Üstün et al., 2016). Thus, this area in the field of environmental health is well-established.

As a result of this general one-way focus, and because of the fact that a public health crisis impacting the movement of people and goods on such a large scale has not happened in recent history, there is a gap in the literature in regard to assessing human health effects on the environment, thus limiting our ability to assess the effects of the COVID-19 pandemic on the environment. As a result, the main research question explored by this book is: Within the context of the COVID-19 pandemic, how can the impacts of human health on the environment be organized in a way that will help further in-depth research and encourage a more integrated, fluid approach to solving issues within the field of environmental health?

Therefore, the aim of this research is to work towards closing the aforementioned knowledge gap regarding the connections between the environment and public health (referred to hereafter as "the environment-public health knowledge gap") by developing a framework that can be used to assess the impacts of human health and a health crisis response on the natural environment. This framework is informed by a review of emerging literature on the documented environmental effects of the COVID-19 pandemic in addition to existing literature on environmental impacts of the health care sector.

1.3   Literature Review

It is clear that there is an abundance of research on the impacts of the environment on human health. However, it is apparent that there is a gap in the literature on possible impacts flowing in the opposite direction. Less attention and research have been devoted to understanding the impacts of public health crises and human health impacts in general on the natural environment. Much of the existing literature on this topic currently focuses on extremely specific effects from medical responses and outputs from the health care sector. For example, using the 2009 influenza pandemic as a case study, Singer (2018) evaluated possible environmental effects of the usage of antivirals and antibiotics, which are released into natural bodies of water in a biologically active form through the disposal of human waste into sewage systems. Possible risks included the inhibition of vital microorganisms in wastewater systems and the loss of marine life in river ecosystems. Singer et al. (2011) assessed the ecotoxicological risks of a pandemic medical response in regard to water system health, concluding that a moderate to severe pandemic could affect eutrophication in river ecosystems and contaminate drinking water sources.

With respect to pollution and other environmental impacts from the health care sector, Allen et al. (1986), Walker and Cooper (1992), and Singh and Prakash (2007) assessed toxic air pollution arising from medical waste incineration and the consequences of these releases. Manzoor and Sharma (2019) summarized and discussed the negative effects of inadequate biomedical waste disposal on air, water, and soil quality. Tsakona et al. (2006) examined different categories of hospital waste throughout the entire waste management process, concluding that improvements could be made at every stage in order to lessen environmental impacts. Therefore, a substantial portion of existing literature does focus on assessing the impacts of waste from the health care sector.

Eckelman and Sherman (2016) widened this lens by performing an economic input-output life cycle assessment (EIOLCA) to assess the environmental impacts of the U.S. health care system. This study illustrated some of the more complex ways that human health processes interact with the environment by quantifying life cycle emissions to air, water, and soil and looking at impacts in categories such as global warming, ozone depletion, and acidification (Eckelman & Sherman, 2016). The use of a broader perspective will be crucial to understanding the reverberating effects that COVID-19 will continue to have on the environment as a large-scale natural experiment.

Following the pandemic's medical and socio-economic response from governments around the world, documented effects on various aspects of the environment were quickly observed. One of the primary impacts studied since the beginning of the pandemic was the short-term reduction in traffic-related air pollution in areas of Italy, Spain, France, China, and the United States, with some regions reporting significantly lower nitrogen dioxide (NO_2) levels compared to levels during the same period in 2019 (Muhammad et al., 2020; Zambrano-Monserrate et al., 2020). In China, lower industrial energy combustion from reduced economic activity during its lockdown indicated a significant reduction in greenhouse gas emissions compared to the same period in 2019 (Wang & Su, 2020). Additionally, reductions in recreational and industrial activity contributed to improved water quality in the Venice Lagoon and in rivers in India (Arora et al., 2020; Braga et al., 2020; Lokhandwala & Gautam, 2020).

Not all impacts have been positive. In regard to waste, effects have been complex due to the fact that the pandemic has caused an increase in demand for disposable goods while also weakening economies, which has led to a reduction in consumption. While plastic demand in certain sectors originally declined, there was simultaneously an increase in medical waste from the greater usage of protective equipment and an increase in single-use plastic waste from food delivery (Klemeš et al., 2020).

Thus, as a natural experiment of a massive scale, COVID-19 is exposing effects that may have been hidden and is providing the opportunity to assess a vast number of environmental impacts that can stem from a public health crisis and response. Overall, our understanding of these effects has been disjointed at best, and as governments and communities continue to respond and adapt to this public health crisis, the events that are unfolding will continue to have profound impacts on our environment. As a result, developing an organized framework to assess these impacts will aid in informing future research that will help close the environment-public health knowledge gap. The aim is to additionally aid researchers and leaders in preparing better for the future, especially as warming climate trends and greater extreme weather events continue to worsen the impacts of infectious diseases (Patz et al., 2005).

Today, there are already existing frameworks for evaluating environmental impacts from various processes. In the United States, under the National Environmental Policy Act (NEPA), federal agencies are required to take environmental considerations into their decision-making process by preparing detailed reports called Environmental Assessments (EA) and Environmental Impact Statements (EIS) (U.S. Environmental Protection Agency [EPA], 2013). These fall under what the United Nations Environment Programme (UNEP) categorizes as Environmental Impact Assessments (EIA), a type of tool used to evaluate environmental, social, and economic impacts of a specific project prior to its implementation (Convention on Biological Diversity, 2010). In contrast, a Strategic Environmental Assessment (SEA) is used in the more proactive process of evaluating the environmental impacts of proposed policies, plans, or programs from a broader perspective focused on ensuring sustainability (Convention on Biological Diversity, 2010). Life Cycle Analysis (LCA) is another method of impact analysis that is used to quantify and assess the total life cycle effects of a product or activity from the cradle to the grave. "ReCiPe" is a relevant LCA method developed partially by the Dutch government that uses environmental midpoint and endpoint impact categories (National Institute for Public Health and the Environment, 2018). While these existing tools are useful for assessing specific projects or policy considerations and were a source of inspiration for the research conducted in this paper, they are not easily adaptable to use for assessing larger-scale human health and health crisis response impacts on the environment.

In the wake of COVID-19, few frameworks have been developed in an attempt to understand aspects of the global public health response. Bates et al. (2020) categorized the pandemic and its subsequent lockdown efforts as a "Global Human Confinement Experiment," whereby rapid and widespread restrictions on human mobility provided the opportunity to study the impacts of these events on biodiversity and conservation. Cheval et al. (2020) developed a spaciotemporal framework for categorizing the various effects of the COVID-19 pandemic on different scales. However, even as researchers are developing methods for assessing the consequences of COVID-19, the aforementioned research gap in the field of environment and public health has left us with few robust tools for comprehensively understanding the wide range of impacts that can result from human health and a health crisis response. For this reason, this study aims to contribute to a better understanding of these effects by using the COVID-19 pandemic to inform the development of a framework that can be used to assess the impacts of a human health crisis on the environment.

1.4   Research Design and Methods

The method used in this research is qualitative review and analysis through a comprehensive literature review of secondary data. In Chapter 4, this research is supported by quantitative analysis of emerging data trends. Through an inductive process, a theoretical framework was designed and created, informed by a review of emerging literature on the documented environmental effects of the COVID-19 pandemic and existing literature on environmental impacts of the health care sector. The purpose of this framework is to assess the impacts of human health on the environment within the context of the COVID-19 pandemic as a global natural experiment. Data was obtained by searching appropriate databases such as Google Scholar, PubMed Central, ScienceDirect, Web of Science, ProQuest, and Scopus. Sources from international organizations such as the WHO and the Centers for Disease Control and Prevention (CDC) are utilized as well. Additional data on the COVID-19 pandemic was obtained from reputable news sources such as the *New York Times* due to the fact that the crisis occurred concurrently with this study.

1.5 Organization

The methods for this study are discussed in depth in Chapter 2, with an explanation of the theoretical framework created for this study and a description of the inductive process used to conduct a literature review, select appropriate impacts, and populate the framework. The results of this review are presented in Chapter 3 and are organized by how they fit into the developed framework. In Chapter 4, the applicability of this framework is "tested" through two case studies, which are used to demonstrate the framework in action, determine its transferability and scalability, and analyze its strengths and weaknesses (Note: The use of the word "tested" in this study is used tentatively due to the fact that this book is based more on theoretical research rather than empirical work. The findings of this study come primarily from observation rather than rigorous testing). The first case study application uses the framework to catalogue the environmental effects of the 2003 Severe Acute Respiratory Syndrome (SARS) outbreak to explore whether the it is applicable for use in analyzing human health crises other than COVID-19. The second case study uses the framework to catalog the environmental effects of the COVID-19 pandemic in New York City to assess whether the tool can be scaled down to focus on a more specific geographic region. Chapter 5 presents a discussion of the primary findings from the literature reviews for Chapters 3 and 4, implications of the research, limitations of the study, future areas for exploration, and the conclusion.

Chapter 2: Methods

2.1 Introduction

The purpose of this research was to develop a framework that could be used to categorize the impacts of a human health crisis on the environment. Because the COVID-19 pandemic has had unprecedented effects on human activity within the past year, it has acted as a global natural experiment, with most of the human population affected in one way or another. During this time, new information and research began to emerge every day in relation to the multitude of effects that COVID-19 was having on various aspects of life, including the environment. In order to capture this emerging data, this study conducted a comprehensive review of both emerging literature about the environmental effects of COVID-19 and some of the existing human health impacts on the environment. The review was accomplished through the use of numerous scholarly websites such as Google Scholar, PubMed Central, ScienceDirect, Web of Science, ProQuest, and Scopus. Sources from national and international organizations such as the CDC, the WHO, and the United Nations (UN) were utilized to obtain official public health guidance and information. Additional data on the effects of the COVID-19 pandemic were obtained from reputable news sources due to the fact that they provided up to date information on emerging effects occurring as the research was being conducted.

Once all of the preliminary research on COVID-19 and existing human health impacts on the environment was consolidated and reviewed, a theoretical framework was developed based on available data through inductive reasoning. The findings of the review and the populated framework are presented in Chapter 3. The framework was designed to be categorical, allowing for the differentiation between both the types of impacts and the general phases in which these effects were occurring. The aim is that this tool will help close the environment-public health knowledge gap and be useful in helping communities understand how a public health crisis may be impacting the environment they live in.

After the framework was established and populated using the COVID-19 pandemic and its environmental effects, it was necessary to find a way to test for and examine its transferability and scalability to other human health crises. It is important to note that within the context of this study, the idea of testing the framework refers to finding a way to apply it, not empirically test it, due to its theoretical nature. Two case studies were conducted for this purpose. The first was an analysis of the 2003 SARS outbreak concentrated primarily in China and some of its neighboring countries. Guided by the established framework and its impact categories, a literature review was carried out on this outbreak to examine the framework's value for use in a completely separate public health crisis. A second case study was then conducted using the same method on New York City's experience with COVID-19 as the original American epicenter of the virus. The purpose of this second case study was to determine the scalability of the framework and determine its usefulness at a more condensed geographical scale rather than a global perspective.

This case study included the only quantitative analysis performed in this research. Because it focused on trends at a more granular level, residential waste collection data was obtained to more fully analyze waste trends that were being reported on in the news. This quantitative work utilized monthly data from the New York City Department of Sanitation (DSNY) for the years of 2015 to 2020 and focused on the waste categories of metal, glass, and plastic (MGP), paper, refuse, and organics. Using excel, data was combined for the years of 2015 to 2019 to find a five-year average for monthly collection trends. The percentage change between these averages and their corresponding months of 2020 was then calculated to determine how much New York City's residential waste trends for the past year have differed in comparison to previous years.

The findings for the two case studies are presented in Chapter 4. Based on the experience of applying the framework, Chapter 5 includes a discussion of findings from Chapters 3 and 4, implications of the framework, limitations of the research, areas for future exploration, and the conclusion.

2.2   Framework

The theoretical framework developed by this research is comprised of five nested half-rings (referred to hereafter as "rings") based on each perceived impact stage of a human health crisis and five main environmental impact categories. These categories were inductively formed through a review of the emerging literature on COVID-19 and inspired by already-established environmental impact frameworks such as EIS and ReCiPe. The structure of the diagram is presented as a half-circle to symbolize the idea that the effects catalogued are not comprehensive and are meant to be a starting point—there is room for expansion and improvement upon this framework.

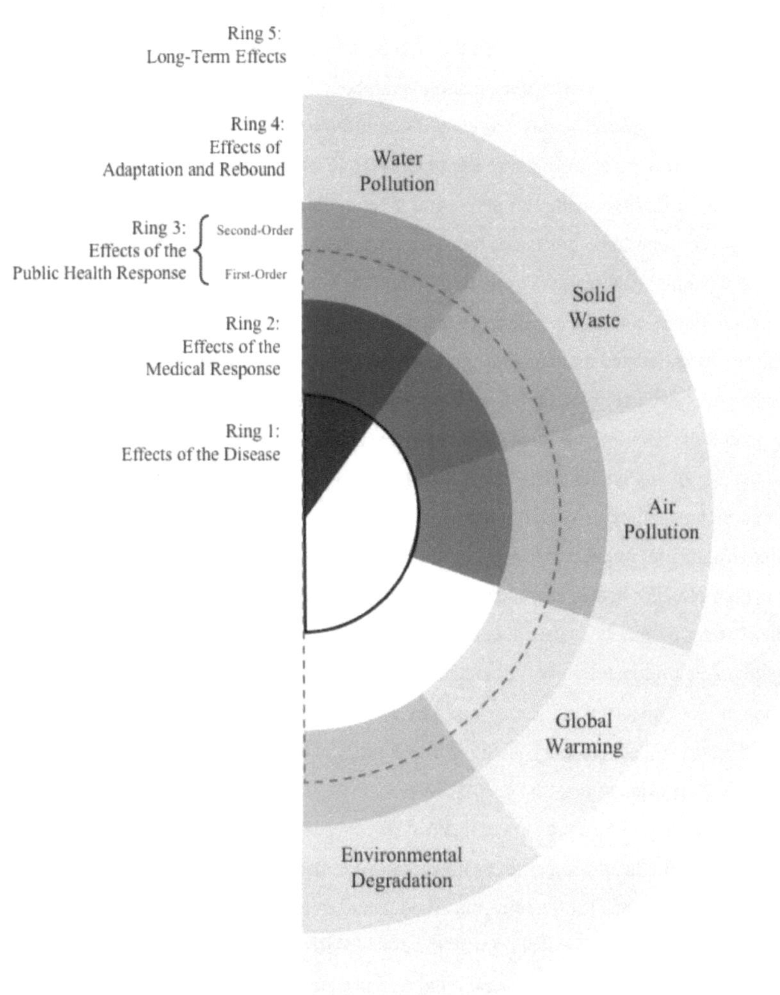

Figure 1. A theoretical framework developed for assessing the impact of a human health crisis on the environment. The framework is comprised of five categories: water pollution, solid waste, air pollution, global warming, and environmental degradation. These impact categories extend through five rings, which represent the effects of the varying stages of a human health crisis over time: the health issue, the medical response, the public health response, adaptation and rebound, and long-term impacts.

2.3   Health Crisis Impact Stages

The five main stages of effects stemming from a human health crisis are as follows: the effects of the health issue or disease itself, the effects of the medical response, the effects of the public health response, the effects of adaptation and rebound, and long-term effects. The establishment of these impact stages was carried out through inductive reasoning based on a review of literature on the emerging impacts of COVID-19 as well as existing impacts of human health issues on the environment. The purpose of creating these categories was to provide a way to differentiate between how effects can happen over time as a result of different human responses to a public health crisis. In this framework, the rings are intertwined with the environmental impact categories, which are discussed in depth below.

The first ring, located in the center of the framework, corresponds to the effects of the health issue or disease itself. While the environmental impacts of a disease or ailment aren't easily apparent, the decision was made to include this category due to the fact that it is the central-most part of any health crisis. For this reason, it was worth looking into in order to broaden our understanding of what it means for human health to impact the environment. The primary environmental impacts discussed in this category are related to water, whereby viral loading in natural water bodies can occur. For this ring specifically, the term "water impacts" rather than "water pollution" is used due to the fact that the existence of a virus or source of illness within a natural water body is not technically thought of as "pollution." In general, this ring embodies any impacts of a disease caused by a virus or bacteria on natural life. Water impacts is the only impact category included in this ring due to the fact that within the literature thus far, there is only documentation of SARS-CoV-2 being detected within water systems.

The second ring corresponds to the medical response to a human health crisis, while the third covers the public health response. Following the coronavirus outbreak, Yang et al. (2020) proposed recommendations for the prevention and management of future coronavirus outbreaks based off of China's experience dealing with the 2003 SARS outbreak and COVID-19. These recommendations fell into four categories: rapid response, treatment, reducing viral transmission, and prevention. For the purpose of this research, this paper differentiates between the medical and public health response to COVID-19, with Ring 2 covering the categories of rapid response and treatment and Ring 3 covering the categories of reduction of viral transmission and prevention. It is important to note that the medical response to the pandemic is inherently encompassed by the larger, accompanying public health response due to the fact that the treatment of an infection and preventing its transmission to others go hand-in-hand. Differentiating between the two, however, allows for a more organized examination of the policies and precautions being taken in healthcare facilities in order to detect and treat the disease.

Therefore, while these rings overlap, Ring 2 primarily focuses on environmental impacts that stem from the detection and treatment of the infection in health care settings and the medical precautions associated with it. Ring 3 focuses on the broader public health policies put in place to reduce the transmission of the disease and prevent its resurgence in the future. Ring 3 is also the only impact stage that is sub-divided into first- and second-order impacts, which denote the consequential succession of environmental impacts in response to public health policies and act as a further way to organize and define this ring, which produced by far the most results out of all impact stages. The inductive review of the literature determined that the three main environmental impact categories associated with the medical response are water pollution, solid waste, and air pollution. This is largely due to the fact that this framework aims to account for medical response effects that directly impact the environment or exacerbate existing impacts of the health care sector. In relation to this focus, the impact categories of global warming and environmental degradation are too far removed from these direct impacts and are thus not included in this impact stage. This is more fully discussed in Ring 2 in Chapter 3. Ring 3, on the other hand, is associated with all five impact categories, all of which are described in depth below.

Ring 4 corresponds to the effects of society's adaptation to and rebound from a human health crisis. This ring considers the effects of adaptation to a human health crisis should it become long-term, much like COVID-19 has. It also looks at the way a society comes back from a human health crisis once it is declared over. The idea of rebounding refers to the impacts that result from the removal of public health policies and measures implemented to prevent the spread of a disease. This impact stage is a bit broader than the previous categories discussed, but it was necessary to include based on how COVID-19 has affected society throughout the past year. Rather than shutting everything down for a short period of time before removing all public health restrictions with the disappearance of the disease, COVID-19 has remained a part of life for over a year, which has resulted in society slowly adapting to it and governments loosening restraints in stages. This ring is associated with all five environmental impact categories as well.

The fifth ring refers to the long-term changes that come out of the period of adaptation and rebound. COVID-19 has taught society to rethink almost every aspect of how everyday life is conducted and organized, and as people have adapted to it, there is indication from the literature that some changes brought on by the pandemic may become either long-term or permanent. This ring is the only ring that is not split into the five environmental impact categories due to the fact that these long-term effects are broad and abstract, and they have the potential to influence numerous aspects of the natural environment.

2.4   Environmental Impact Categories

The five environmental impact categories established by this research are as follows: water pollution, solid waste, air pollution, global warming, and environmental degradation. The establishment of these categories was achieved through inductive reasoning based on a review of the available literature. The aim is that these categories will be useful for classifying impacts from human health issues as they emerge during a crisis in the future.

The first category of water pollution primarily encompasses effects on natural water bodies that are linked to a health crisis and its ensuing medical and public health responses. The review of the literature gathered for this research revealed that numerous aspects of a human health crisis can affect natural bodies of water. These impacts stem largely from viral loading, disinfectant and antiviral pollution, and reduced human activity in natural areas, all of which are discussed in depth in Chapter 3. This is the only category that stretches through each impact stage of the framework. Ring 1 refers to it as "water impacts," while the other five impact stages use the term "water pollution." For the sake of ease, the overall category is called water pollution.

The second environmental impact category is solid waste. This category accounts for changes in quantities of solid waste types that result from a human health crisis. The review of the literature determined that the medical and public health responses to a crisis (as well as the adaptation and rebound period into the long-term) can have pronounced effects on waste streams around the world, including recyclables, refuse, and organic materials. Much of these changes are related to the need for disposability and changes in human behavior. This impact category is included in Rings 2 through 5.

The third category is air pollution, which refers to changes in atmospheric pollutants such as nitrogen oxides (NO_x, which is a group of pollutants that includes nitrogen dioxide (NO_2)), particulate matter (both $PM_{2.5}$ and PM_{10}), carbon monoxide (CO), sulfur dioxide (SO_2), and ground-level ozone (O_3). Key findings from the literature showed that air pollution can arise from hazardous medical waste disposal through incineration, while public health policies aimed at limiting travel and human interaction (in order to quell the spread of germs) can have a significant short-term impact on numerous air pollutants. This category can be found in Rings 2 through 5, and it does not refer to carbon dioxide (CO_2) due to the fact that it is not a criteria air pollutant according to the EPA (EPA, 2014). CO_2 is instead covered by the fourth environmental impact category, global warming, for the role that it plays as a greenhouse gas in changing the greenhouse effect on Earth, which can lead to climate change through either warming or cooling. Changes in CO_2 levels arose in conjunction with changes in air pollutants as a result of public health policies, though they were short-lived. Overall, this category spans Rings 3 through 5.

The final category is called environmental degradation, and it encompasses the multitude of harmful impacts that can occur towards natural ecosystems beyond that of the pre-existing impacts of health care systems (discussed in Eckelman & Sherman, 2016). Effects such as reduced noise pollution, disinfectant poisoning of wild animals, and a lack of environmental monitoring observed within the literature stemmed from the varied ways in which humans have interacted with the environment throughout the various stages of the pandemic. This area touches on ideas such as conservation and biodiversity protection, and its breadth has implications for further categorization in the future. This category spans Rings 3 through 5.

Chapter 3: Populating a Framework

3.1 Ring 1: Effects of the Health Issue

3.1.1 Introduction

Ring 1 examines the potential effects of a health problem or disease itself on the environment within the context of the observed and expected effects of SARS-CoV-2. Overall, the literature has documented one main effect on the natural environment in this impact stage, along with two other notable effects that do not fit into the scope of this framework but are mentioned for their relevance. The main environmental impact category explored in this section is water impacts. Ring 1 is the only impact stage in this framework that refers to this category as "water impacts" rather than "water pollution" due to the fact that the viral presence of a disease is not typically considered a traditional source of pollution—it is more of a presence. The main water impact observed is that SARS-CoV-2 has been found in wastewater systems. Two other notable effects explored as a result of the health issue itself are human mortality and reverse zoonotic transmission. These topics are related to humans and other forms of life in captivity and therefore do not fully fit into the structure of the framework.

3.1.2 Water Impacts: The Persistence of SARS-CoV-2 in Wastewater

In recent years, many viruses have been detected in the stools and urine of infected individuals, and research has reported the possible presence of enveloped viruses such as a coronavirus in wastewater sewage systems (Race et al., 2020). This resulted in increased vigilance in the scientific community over the likelihood of SARS-CoV-2 persisting in wastewater. Since the beginning of the COVID-19 pandemic, detection of SARS-CoV-2 has been confirmed: In April, researchers reported the first detection of this virus in wastewater in Australia determined through RNA sequencing (Ahmed et al., 2020). In addition, SARS-CoV-2 was detected in the stools of COVID-19 patients and sewage systems. As a result, there is a possibility for transmission of the virus through contaminated drinking water and other sources if it is left untreated in sewage (Heller et al., 2020; Gwenzi, 2020; Bhowmick et al., 2020). For this reason, proper wastewater management and sanitation are important in preventing the further spread of SARS-CoV-2.

3.1.3 Human Mortality

Though humans and human activity are often considered to be separate from nature, people are inherently a part of the environment as living organisms. For this reason, though this framework is assessing impacts of human health crises on the environment and is not structured to account for this impact, it is still important to acknowledge the loss of life that is occurring as a result of the COVID-19 pandemic. As of April 16th, 2021, 139 million cases have been recorded worldwide and over 2.9 million individuals have died (JHU CSSE, 2021). Because of its severity, the pandemic is likely to fundamentally change the way humans approach health crises in the future.

3.1.4   *Reverse Zoonotic Transmission: Instances of SARS-CoV-2 in Animals*

A second impact that the virus is having on lifeforms is transmission of the virus from humans to other species. In 2020, SARS-CoV-2 was thought to have originated from a seafood and wet animal wholesale market in Wuhan, Hubei Province, China, after local health facilities reported groups of patients with symptoms of pneumonia in December 2019 (Zhu et al., 2020). In recent months, however, there has been discourse over whether this market was actually the source or rather just the site of a super-spreader event (Ewe, 2020). It remains, however, that SARS-CoV-2 is a zoonotic disease most likely originating from bats (Zhou et al., 2020). As a source of previous coronaviruses, researchers believe that bats possibly transmitted SARS-CoV-2 to another animal before it was transmitted to humans.

Following COVID-19's spread around the globe, there have also been reports of transmission of the disease back to animals through "reverse zoonosis," a process that is not well-researched but has been documented across the world in the past (Messenger et al., 2014). According to the CDC, there have been reports of animals becoming infected worldwide, including cats and dogs, several lions and tigers in a New York City Zoo, and mink in Europe and the United States (CDC, 2020a). In most cases, these animals are thought to have contracted the virus after being exposed to infected humans, and there is currently little evidence that animals are significantly transmitting SARS-CoV-2 to people (CDC, 2020a). Beyond this, other studies have concluded that certain animals may be susceptible to contracting SARS-CoV-2. Since it is established that SARS-CoV-2 can enter water systems, there is a chance that aquatic mammals (dolphins and whales in particular) are at risk of developing COVID-19 due to their susceptibility to contracting viral pneumonia (Nabi & Khan, 2020). Thus far, it appears that most animals infected are either domesticated or have been in the care of humans. Because most cases of reverse zoonosis were documented in animals in captivity, this is not considered a natural impact, but it is included for its relevance.

3.1.5 *Summary*

When considering the effects of an actual disease outbreak itself, the most stunning effects have clearly been those on human life. Traditional thought on environmental impacts however, often concerns damage to aspects of nature such as air, water, and wildlife. As a result, the impacts of human mortality and reverse zoonotic transmission among animals exposed to humans explored within this section can be viewed as unique categories of impact that do not fall under this framework but are still relevant due to their significant impacts on humans and other species. When these effects are removed from the process of populating this framework, the main environmental category remaining concerns impacts on water systems. For this ring, the only environmental impact category populated by an analysis of the COVID-19 pandemic is consequently water impacts. This is due to the fact that at the time this research was conducted, the literature only documented that SARS-CoV-2 had been detected in water compartments.

3.2 Ring 2: Effects of the Medical Response

3.2.1 *Introduction*

It is crucial to understand that the environmental impacts resulting from the COVID-19 pandemic must be understood within the greater context of the impacts that health care systems already inflict on the environment. As discussed in Chapter 2, there is already a significant amount of literature published related to existing health care-related impacts on the environment. Through their economic life cycle assessment of the US healthcare sector, Eckelman and Sherman (2016) found that this sector is responsible for significant impacts on air quality through acid rain, greenhouse gas emissions, smog formation, criteria air pollutants, stratospheric ozone depletion, and both carcinogenic and non-carcinogenic air toxins. Manzoor and Sharma (2019) reviewed the impacts of biomedical waste on different aspects of the natural environment, concluding that biomedical waste can have serious impacts on water, soil quality, and air quality. Other studies have established that medical waste incineration ejects toxic heavy metals into the air and contributes to air pollution (Allen et al., 1986; Singh & Prakash, 2007). The purpose of this section is to examine how the medical response to COVID-19 fits into the environmental impacts of the health care sector and how it may be exacerbating certain aspects of it.

As discussed in Chapter 2, Yang et al. (2020) proposes four main categories of recommendations for the future management of coronavirus outbreaks or similar events: rapid response, treatment, reducing viral transmission, and prevention. Though the medical response to a health crisis is inherently encompassed by a larger public health response due to the fact that treatment and prevention of transmission are closely related, it is necessary to differentiate between the two in order to more closely focus on the environmental impacts that stem from the detection and treatment of the infection, as well as medical precautions taken in health care facilities. Overall, the medical response to COVID-19 (covered by Ring 2) has encompassed rapid response, detection measures, and treatment.

3.2.2 *Water Pollution*

The medical response to COVID-19 has largely included the use of existing antivirals and other medications to help treat the disease as countries have struggled to cope with determining the best method of treatment (Mitjà & Clotet, 2020). Within the literature, it is established that when used, antivirals are released in high quantities into wastewater through the disposal of human waste and bodily fluids. This poses possible environmental risks to various water systems, including the inhibition of microorganisms in wastewater systems and harm to marine life in river ecosystems (Singer, 2018; Singer et al., 2011, Sanderson et al., 2004, Nannou et al., 2020). In response to COVID-19, multiple forms of antiviral treatments are being tested through clinical trials as possible forms of therapy for the disease. Some antivirals being tested for use in treating COVID-19 show low potential for ecotoxicological characteristics, while others demonstrate higher potential due to the fact that antivirals are often excreted as unchanged compounds that are highly bioactive. For example, the antiviral lopinavir has a high bioaccumulation potential in wastewater streams and could possibly pose an ecotoxicological risk (Race et al., 2020). Other anti-malarial drugs such as chloroquine and hydroxychloroquine, which were also being tested to determine if they have effective antiviral properties, pose a risk to water sources and should be classified as harmful to aquatic organisms (Race et al., 2020). These drugs, however, have not been approved for use in treatment and are therefore not included in the population of this framework.

A second main effect of the medical response to COVID-19 on water quality stems from the use of disinfectant in hospitals and other health facilities in order to protect health care workers and prevent the transmission of the virus. Official guidelines from the CDC for ensuring the cleanliness of health care facilities include using an EPA-registered hospital disinfectant and established sterilization methods to clean surfaces and patient-care devices (CDC, 2019). While disinfectant is a crucial part of containing and preventing the spread of COVID-19 in hospitals and beyond, the use of these substances is harmful to aquatic organisms. Disinfectant can end up in water systems such as lakes through runoff and through wastewater sewage systems. In particular, chlorine disinfectants pose a risk to plants and animals because they can damage their cells and proteins and can bond with other compounds in a body of water to form highly ecotoxic by-products (Zhang et al., 2020).

3.2.3 Solid Waste

The medical response to COVID-19 is also having pronounced effects on the waste sector, leading to increased medical waste from greater personal protective equipment (PPE) and medical supply usage. Due to rising demand earlier this year, there was a severe risk of a PPE shortage as countries and health care systems struggled to cope with the pandemic. This led to the WHO calling on industries and governments to increase the manufacturing of PPE by 40 percent to meet global demand and maintain supply chains (WHO, 2020). This increase in PPE usage has been a crucial part of treating COVID-19 patients and stopping the spread, but it has also led to a dramatic increase in the generation of medical waste. This is a direct impact of treatment due to the fact that standard and transmission-based precautions are recommended in treating or encountering patients with COVID-19. Precautions include wearing eye protection such as a face shield or goggles, face masks, N95 or higher respirators, gloves, and gowns to prevent transmission (CDC, 2020b). While some PPE can be reused, such as certain eye protection, gowns, and respirators, other PPE is often disposed of after use, indicating that disposability is crucial to sanitation and hygiene. This uptick in the generation of biomedical hazardous waste has implications for the environment.

Studies are indicating that hospitals are also generating larger amounts of medical waste due to the influx of patients being treated with COVID-19. In Jordan, the average rate of medical waste generated per day in hospitals from treating COVID-19 increased by over tenfold compared to the average waste generation rate during regular periods (Abu-Qdais et al., 2020). In Hubei Province, China, the generation of medical waste increased by 370 percent, with a high proportion of this being made up of plastics (Klemeš et al., 2020). In Bangladesh, at least 14,500 tonnes of waste from health care activities was generated in April due to COVID-19, with an average of 206 tonnes of medical waste being produced per day in Dhaka (Rahman et al., 2020).

Overall, it is estimated that the pandemic could result in the monthly consumption and waste of 129 billion face masks and 65 billion gloves (Prata et al., 2020).

With this greater pressure on waste streams around the world, there is also an increased likelihood that much of this waste will be disposed of improperly, and there is anecdotal evidence that PPE is emerging in greater quantities in the natural environment. Around the world, discarded PPE is showing up on beaches and in other natural places (Silva et al., 2020; Winters, 2020). As infectious litter made of single-use plastic, these hazardous waste materials are causing increased contamination in the environment while also contributing to the plastic crisis. These materials also have the ability to pervade throughout the entire globe due to environmental processes, and they eventually break down into microplastics that exist in the natural environment for hundreds of years (Prata et al., 2020).

3.2.4 Air Pollution

The disposal of increased quantities of medical waste due to the COVID-19 pandemic has led to a general increase in hospital waste incineration. Due to the high infectivity risk of medical waste generated during the COVID-19 pandemic, incineration is considered the best method of disposal in order to prevent transmission from untreated waste (Ma et al., 2020). While some hospital waste incineration plants weren't originally operating at peak capacity prior to the pandemic, the usage and disposal of medical waste during this time has brought many plants to full capacity. At the beginning of the pandemic in Wuhan, China, medical waste increased from the normal level of 40 tonnes per day to a peak of 240 tonnes per day, which exceeded the maximum incineration capacity of 49 tonnes per day (Klemeš et al., 2020). As waste incineration is responsible for ejecting heavy metals and other toxic substances into the air, it can therefore be assumed that the medical response to COVID-19 has had pronounced effects on air quality.

Another factor to consider is the dominant method of disposal of medical waste in different countries around the world. While some countries and facilities have the technology and resources to incinerate waste with the best techniques, others do not, which could lead to the release of toxic substances such as polychlorinated dibenzodioxins (PCDD) and polychlorinated dibenzofurans (PCDF) in high concentrations through improper burning. Furthermore, other countries have resorted to burning hazardous waste through methods of open pit burning, which additionally contributes to air pollution (UNEP, 2020). Understanding and tracking the differing methods of disposal for medical waste associated with COVID-19 is therefore important to understanding the environmental impacts that the pandemic's medical response is having on air quality.

3.2.5 Summary

Through this section, it is established that effects on water pollution, waste, and air pollution are three main impact categories to consider when assessing how a health crisis like the COVID-19 pandemic can affect the natural environment. The main sources of water pollution that pose a risk are antiviral treatments and disinfectants. Evidence shows that antivirals can make their way into water systems through the human excretion of bodily fluids, and disinfectants used to sanitize health care facilities may end up in the natural environment through runoff or wastewater systems. Both sources of pollution can have a negative effect on aquatic organisms. Neither of these effects have been directly observed during the pandemic, but documented existing impacts of medical practices show that this is possible. For this reason, this is worth monitoring at a time when these treatments and products are being used.

Solid waste effects related to the pandemic have stemmed from a large increase in the demand for and use of PPE as a protective measure for health care workers. Cities observed a large increase in medical waste generation from their medical facilities, with much of the increase coming from single-use plastic items. This evidence was paired with anecdotal observations of greater amounts of disposable PPE emerging within natural areas due to improper disposal. Because this evidence is largely anecdotal and this impact cannot be traced specifically to the aspects of the medical response or public health response directly, environmental degradation is not included as a category within this impact stage of the framework.

Air pollution impacts from the global medical response include an increase in the emissions of toxic air pollutants due to both proper and improper sanitary disposal of medical waste through incineration or open pit burning. Overall, the effects observed in this section act as a supplement to literature on existing impacts of medical treatment and the health care sector on the environment. It is not meant to encompass all impacts but rather to highlight some of the main ways in which the concentrated medical response to COVID-19 may be exacerbating certain effects with health care facilities working at capacity.

3.3 Ring 3: Effects of the Public Health Response

3.3.1 Introduction

In comparison to Ring 2, the third impact stage encompasses the broader public health response that has occurred during the COVID-19 pandemic. Whereas the medical response has been characterized by reactive measures (rapid response, detection, and treatment), the public health response can be characterized by proactive measures. Yang et al. (2020) describes reducing viral transmission and further prevention as two other crucial categories for dealing with coronavirus outbreaks. These two categories of action and their associated impacts will be covered within this ring as they are proactive public health measures. In addition, due to the fact that the public health response to COVID-19 has been so extensive, the magnitude of its effects in terms of first-order and second-order impacts will be considered, with first-order impacts encompassing direct effects of public health policies and second-order impacts referring to indirect impacts that are one degree of magnitude removed from these policies. This section first provides a summary of the public health response to COVID-19 and some of its consequences followed by a summary of the environmental impacts organized by impact category.

3.3.2 Understanding the Public Health Response to COVID-19

Since the novel coronavirus proliferated around the world, social distancing and lockdown measures such as school closures, travel bans, and quarantine have continuously been imposed in various countries (Dunford et al., 2020; Salcedo et al., 2020). One of the most consequential public health policies has been the travel ban. Beginning in March, numerous countries decided to restrict travel from other countries excluding their own citizens, including the United States, Canada, Australia, Germany, and many others. The European Union also restricted non-essential travel within the region for at least 30 days (O'Hare & Hardingham-Gill, 2020, Salcedo et al., 2020). One main result of these restrictions was the steep decline in air travel. In April of 2020, the number of people flying dropped by 96 percent to a 10-year low, causing airlines to cut 71 percent of their capacity (Wallace, 2020). In general, daily aviation activity declined by an average of 75 percent. Because air travel requires a massive amount of fuel, these declines resulted in a short-term decline of 60 percent in greenhouse gas emissions from the aviation sector (Le Quéré et al., 2020a).

A second significant type of public health policy implemented was the lockdown order, which forced schools, businesses, and workplaces into closure around the world. By the end of

March, over 100 national governments around the world had ordered a lockdown or partial lockdown whereby most or all non-essential internal movement was restricted. One of the most severe orders came in Italy, one of the countries hardest hit originally by the virus. Citizens were only allowed to leave their houses for work or health reasons, a 6 p.m. curfew was imposed, and schools, universities, cinemas, theaters, gyms, and other public venues were order to close (Borrelli, 2020). Many other countries that did not impose lockdown orders still made recommendations for restricted movement. As a result of these policies, an estimated 4.4 billion people around the world experienced some sort of lockdown (Bates et al., 2020).

The combined travel restrictions and lockdown orders have had rippling effects through-out society. In addition to reducing flights worldwide, lockdown orders reduced all forms of movement and travel. Transport mobility decreased by 54 percent in the US, 89 percent in Spain, 86 percent in Italy, 82 percent in France, 47 percent in Germany, and 70 percent in the United Kingdom, resulting in profound short-term effects on environmental factors (Muhammad et al., 2020). In comparison to mean 2019 emissions, daily global CO_2 emissions decreased by 17 percent at the peak of the lockdown period in April 2020, which was when most people were in confinement. Nearly half of these emissions reductions came from the decline in surface transport (cars, light vehicles, buses and trucks, and national and international shipping), which fell by 36 percent during the same period (Le Quéré et al., 2020a).

In addition to the surface transport and aviation sectors, daily global greenhouse gas emissions at the height of the lockdown period fell by 7.4 percent in the power sector, which accounts for energy conversion for electricity and heat generation. In the industry sector, which comprises of emissions from industrial material production and manufacturing, emissions fell by 19 percent. The public sector, which includes emissions from public buildings and commerce, saw a 21 percent daily decline in CO_2 emissions. Lastly, residential emissions increased by 2.8 percent, likely due to the increased numbers of people staying at home. This only marginally offset the overall decline in emissions (Le Quéré et al., 2020a).

The decrease in transport activity also led to a short-term improvement in certain indicators of air quality. NO_2, one of the main air pollutants emitted to the atmosphere through the combustion of fuel, showed significant declines in cities and regions around the world (Wang & Su, 2020; European Environment Agency [EEA], 2020; Muhammad et al., 2020; Dantas et al., 2020; Kerimray et al., 2020; Zambrano-Monserrate et al., 2020; Lokhandwala & Gautam, 2020;

Helm, 2020). Declines in levels of other air pollutants such as $PM_{2.5}$, PM_{10}, CO, and SO_2 have been less consistent but have still been documented (Dantas et al., 2020; Hamway, 2020; Kerimray et al., 2020; Lokhandwala & Gautam, 2020; Wang & Su, 2020; Zambrano-Monserrate et al., 2020). Ground-level ozone quantities, however, have increased due to the lower ratio of nitrogen oxides in the air (Siciliano et al., 2020; Dantas et al., 2020; Kerimray et al., 2020; Arora et al., 2020). The decrease in industrial activity, human activity, and transport due to lockdown orders also led to noticeable improvements in water quality in certain regions of the world. Improvements stemmed from reductions in human activity and recreation and decreased pollution from decreased industrial activity (Braga et al., 2020; Lokhandwala & Gautam, 2020.) These impacts are discussed in depth below.

Another effect of the lockdown policies combined with travel restrictions was the decline of environmental monitoring. With parks employees remaining at home due to stay-at-home orders, monitoring of natural areas that are crucial to environmental protection and conservation was reduced. The lack of wildlife protection and enforcement presented an opportunity for the increase in environmental degradation, illegal hunting and poaching, and deforestation (Hamwey, 2020; Helm, 2020; López-Feldman et al., 2020). In addition, since many countries rely on ecotourism as a crucial source of revenue for their economy, the rapid decline in this industry and its income had the potential to reduce incentives to protect forests and their biodiversity (López-Feldman, 2020). However, at the same time, some positive environmental aspects were observed during the most intense lockdown periods directly due to the lower interaction of humans with nature. One main effect was the reduction in noise pollution (Arora et al., 2020; Zambrano-Monserrate et al., 2020). Another was the decline in human-induced forest fires in Nepal (Paudel, 2020). This effect is isolated from the climate-change induced wildfires that ravaged the Pacific Northwest of the United States during the summer months of 2020.

Lockdown orders were also responsible for a multitude of impacts on local and national level waste streams. While the extent of the changes occurring to waste flows has yet to be fully assessed, preliminary assessments have contributed to a few stand-out points. (1) There were observed decreases in municipal solid waste. (2) There were changes in household waste disposal and habits. (3) Demand and use of disposable plastic packaging increased. (4) Plastic demand in non-medical and food service sectors decreased due to depressed spending and economic activity. (5) Commercial organic waste increased due to the degradation of unused exports. (6) In general, there has been an increase in plastic waste during the pandemic due to a number of direct public health policies that have altered sustainable waste management policies to limit transmission of the virus. These policies included prohibiting residents from sorting their own waste, banning reusable shopping items such as bags and cups, and postponing zero-waste policies that are aimed at reducing plastic waste (Zambrano-Monserrate et al., 2020; "The Unexpected Environmental Consequences of COVID-19," 2020; Chua, 2020). Plastic waste increased due to behavior choices that changed as people began adjusting to living under a pandemic (Zambrano-Monserrate et al., 2020; Hamwey, 2020; Klemeš et al., 2020; Ragazzi et al., 2020). Many prefer plastic items when ordering food now due to the fact that disposability is associated with sanitation, and because people are under lockdowns and restrictions, many are resorting to ordering more off of the internet, which requires more disposable packaging.

Public health policies regarding community protection are also contributing to the increase in plastic waste. Mask mandates or recommendations have been implemented in countries around the world for the sake of self-protection and the protection of others, as mask usage has been found to possibly reduce infection risk by 85 percent (He & Laurent, 2020). This increase in the usage of masks in everyday life will likely play a role in affecting waste streams around the world. There is also a risk of improper disposal of infectious waste from PPE use leading to the further spread of the virus (Kulkarni & Anantharama, 2020). When disposed of improperly, masks and PPE can end up in the natural environment, and there have been observations of discarded PPE showing up on beaches and in other natural places around the world (Silva et al., 2020; Winters, 2020). This also contributes to the issue of microplastics, which are formed when discarded plastics break down and remain in the environment for long periods of time (Prata et al., 2020).

Social distancing, isolation, and quarantine measures are also being implemented to reduce the transmission of disease among individuals. Recommended by the CDC, social distancing refers to keeping a six-foot distance from other individuals both indoors and outdoors (CDC, 2020c). Policies regarding social distancing have been established and enforced in many communities used in conjunction with other public health measures such as quarantine and isolation. Isolation policies separate individuals who have contracted a contagious disease from people who are not sick. Quarantine separates and restricts people who were exposed to a contagious disease due to the fact that they may become sick after exposure (CDC, 2019).

Another public health policy being implemented is the increase in the use of disinfectant in public areas in order to prevent transmission of the virus. The effects of this practice go hand-in-hand with the previous effects described by the use of disinfectant as a part of the medical response. The CDC recommends using soap and water to clean surfaces before using an EPA-approved disinfectant that is known to kill SARS-CoV-2 (CDC, 2020d). As discussed, the increased usage of disinfectant poses a risk to water bodies through runoff and wastewater systems, where it has the potential to bond with other compounds, form ecotoxic by-products, and harm wildlife (Zhang et al., 2020). It also poses a risk to urban wildlife, with animals at risk of consuming these toxic chemicals and causing their proliferation throughout a local food chain.

Another major part of the coronavirus public health response has been the massive push around the world to develop a vaccine for immunization. By December 2020, numerous countries around the world began to approve the first vaccines aimed at preventing individuals from contracting SARS-CoV-2. The United States approved the Pfizer-BioNTech and Moderna COVID-19 vaccines on December 11th and December 18th, 2020, respectively, through emergency use authorization (U.S. Food and Drug Administration [FDA], 2020a; FDA, 2020b). By February of 2021, the Janssen COVID-19 vaccine (known colloquially as the Johnson & Johnson vaccine) was additionally approved as a third option, though its distribution has since been put on pause (FDA, 2021). While this process will inherently come with waste generation and energy consumption, the widespread distribution of vaccinations could have disparate effects on medical waste disposal, particularly in developing countries where infrastructure is not robust enough to adequately deal with the influx of waste. Vaccination campaigns can lead to the improper dumping of medical waste such as vials, needles, and packaging in pits and other locations ("Addressing Vaccine Waste," 2014). This will be important to consider as COVID-19 vaccinations continue to be developed and distributed around the world.

In addition, buildings and households are being retrofitted with updated heating, ventilation, and air conditioning systems (HVAC) and germicidal UVC light systems that help sterilize and filter indoor air and kill viruses on surfaces (O'Brien, 2020). As the environmental impacts of these proactive measures have not yet been fully assessed, there is a need for further research into these changes as they are increasingly implemented. One can expect that the installment and use of new systems for increased filtration and safety will require greater amounts of energy.

Lastly, due to the fact that SARS-CoV-2 was originally thought to have originated from a "wet" market in Wuhan, China, there has been increased scrutiny surrounding wildlife trade and illegal wildlife trafficking due to the inherent risk of zoonotic diseases being transmitted through these practices. Early in 2020, following the outbreak of SARS-CoV-2, China announced a permanent ban on wildlife trade and consumption, excluding medicinal uses (Gorman, 2020). In addition, it is important to note that wildlife trafficking and crime have detrimental effects on both biodiversity and human health (United Nations Office on Drugs and Crime [UNODC], 2020). Should more of these policies come to the forefront in the coming months, they may have effects on conservation efforts in addition to the protection of human health through the prevented transmission of zoonotic diseases.

3.3.3 *Water Pollution*

In various regions, a first-order effect of public health policies was that natural water bodies saw an improvement in quality due to the reduction of human activities and pollution. With less tourism and recreational activities due to lockdowns and travel restrictions, direct disturbance of important bodies of water declined. Analysis of suspended matter in the lagoon of Venice indicated that the reduction of mobility, tourism, and water traffic during the lockdown in March to April contributed to unprecedented water transparency in city canals (Braga et al., 2020).

Another notable first-order effect is the possible impacts of the use of disinfectants on water bodies and aquatic ecosystems. Throughout the pandemic, disinfectant became an important part of both the medical and the public health response, with governments using crews to disinfect public spaces. As discussed in Ring 2, disinfectants will have adverse effects on water bodies and the ecosystems to which they are home because they are ecotoxic (Zhang et al., 2020). Use of these substances in public spaces poses a risk of these toxic chemicals entering aquatic compartments through runoff and sewage systems.

The main second-order effect observed regarding water pollution and quality is that the reduction of industrial activity during periods of lockdown was linked to a decline in sewage and pollution levels in some instances. Due to the lack of industrial effluents pollution under lockdown, rivers in India such as the Ganga, Cauvery, Sutlej, and Yamuna saw improvements in water quality demonstrated by greater dissolved oxygen levels (Lokhandwala & Gautam, 2020). In addition, surface water quality improved and dissolved oxygen levels increased. This was correlated with reduced disturbance of the waterways due to human activities from tourism, fairs, bathing, and laundry (Arora et al., 2020). While this effect may not have been seen in major water bodies everywhere due to a myriad of other factors, this correlation is still relevant.

3.3.4 Solid Waste

In regard to waste trends, numerous effects related to plastic demand and waste trends were observed in different sectors as a result of public health policies. Some of the first-order effects observed have included changes in municipal solid waste and household waste disposal and habits. Second-order observations include increased demand for and use of disposable plastic packaging, decreased demand for plastic in other sectors, and increased organic waste due to unused exports. The general increase in plastic waste as a result of the pandemic is both a first- and second-order effect due to numerous policies and changes in society. First-order waste effects have stemmed from the direct result of people staying at home due to lockdown orders, while second-order effects have resulted from choices made under lockdown and larger rippling effects throughout the economy.

A significant first-order effect within the waste impact category was the increase in plastic waste due to revised sustainable waste policies. In various countries, differing decisions were made regarding sustainable waste practices out of an abundance of caution for public health. Early on, it was thought that there was a possibility for the transmission of SARS-CoV-2 via reusable materials, and disposable materials were seen as the safest option for buying goods. While this has since been dispelled by emerging research, changes in or postponement of policies such as plastic bag bans have had an impact on the waste stream (Zambrano-Monserrate et al., 2020, Klemeš et al., 2020). Some countries such as the U.S. saw municipalities postponing recycling programs due to the concern of transmission within recycling centers. Other policies such as community waste sorting programs were also affected: In Italy, infected residents were not allowed to sort their own waste due to the fear of transmission of SARS-CoV-2 (Zambrano-Monserrate et al., 2020). Some businesses chose to implement temporary bans on reusable cups or bags, and municipalities overturned or postponed disposable bag bans ("The Unexpected Environmental Consequences of COVID-19," 2020). For example, businesses such as Starbucks began temporarily banning reusable mugs and bags, and multiple state and city governments decided to postpone their plastic bag bans, including New York, Massachusetts, Maine, and

Oregon. Increases in Styrofoam sales were also being seen in the food packaging and health care sectors (Chua, 2020).

Beyond changes to sustainable waste policies, there has also been a general increase in plastic waste due to the widespread usage of face masks as part of both the medical and public health responses. With the increased usage of masks and other PPE aimed at reducing transmission, it is estimated that the pandemic could result in the monthly consumption and waste of 129 billion face masks and 65 billion gloves (Prata et al., 2020).

Changes have also been observed in different countries when it comes to municipal solid waste and household waste streams. During the height of the COVID-19 outbreak in China, municipal solid waste in large and medium cities declined by 30 percent (Klemeš et al). In March 2020 in Trento Italy, the production of MSW was 18.5 percent lower than the March average in the previous 10 years as a result of the lockdown (Ragazzi et al., 2020). The authors note, however, that citizens were likely choosing to accumulate MSW at home instead, postponing transportation. As a result, they predicted a peak in transportation following the easing of lockdown restrictions. Regarding household waste, an increase in demand for the home delivery of goods such as groceries has led to increased organic and inorganic waste generated by households (Zambrano-Monserrate et al., 2020). At the same time, a study conducted in Morocco indicated that household waste declined during the lockdown period in 2020 in comparison to the same period in 2019 (Ouhsine et al., 2020). This disparity is likely due to the fact that numerous social, cultural, and economic factors play a role in household waste generation in communities around the world. Thus far, though household waste estimates have differed under the pandemic, changes are nevertheless being observed, indicating that household waste streams are being influenced by life under the pandemic.

A second crucial part of the public health response, described by Yang et al. (2020) as further prevention, includes the development and distribution of vaccines around the world. In addition to the greater quantities of medical waste that will be created, the widespread distribution and use of vaccines for SARS-CoV-2 may lead to the improper disposal of used syringes and other materials in the environment in certain countries around the world. This is indicated due to observed effects from previous vaccination campaigns and indicates a risk to both the environmental and public health and sanitation ("Addressing Vaccine Waste," 2014).

With the prevalence of lockdown orders implemented at the beginning of the pandemic, numerous second-order effects of widespread public health policies and directives emerged as well. Due to the fact that greater numbers of people were staying home, there was an increased demand for and use of disposable plastic packaging leading to increased plastic waste (Hamwey, 2020; Klemeš et al., 2020; Ragazzi et al., 2020; Zambrano-Montserrate et al., 2020). In many ways, the reasoning for which demand for disposable packaging increased was two-fold: (1) It is commonly thought that sanitation is associated with disposability, and (2) since people were remaining at home, they were ordering more off of the internet, which requires more disposable packaging. While evidence does not suggest that plastics are any safer in comparison to other materials when it comes to transmitting the virus, disposability through single-use plastics has been seen as safer by the general public (Klemeš et al., 2020).

In contrast, during the height of lockdown policies, plastic demand was observed to drop in other economic sectors due to the fact that economic activity was depressed as a result of the pandemic and its consequent lockdown conditions. As a result, plastic demand in non-medical sectors such as the automotive and aviation sectors dropped (Klemeš et al., 2020). The changing dynamics of waste trends seen as a result of economic factors and public health policies present an interesting area for further research.

Lastly, following the heaviest lockdown restrictions, there was an observed increase in organic waste resulting from a reduction in fishery and export levels. According to the United Nations Conference on Trade and Development, cuts in agricultural and fishery exports due to lockdown import restrictions and the decline in the availability of cargo transportation services led to the increased generation of organic waste. Once-normal levels of output for exported goods declined, leading to volumes of goods remaining within countries, unable to be absorbed by domestic markets. As a result, it was reported that food exports in certain areas were left to rot, leading to the compounding environmental effect of greater methane emissions as the food decayed (Hamwey, 2020).

Overall, the public health response has caused significant changes to different waste sectors around the world on both a first and second order of magnitude, necessitating the inclusion of waste as an environmental category within this framework. While some effects can be differentiated through first- and second-order classification, the specifics and quantification of these changes require further in-depth analysis and are beyond the scope of this study.

3.3.5   Air Pollution

As a result of lockdown policies implemented by governments around the world in order to prevent the spread of SARS-CoV-2, individuals stayed at home and limited traveling. During this time, transport mobility decreased heavily all over the world (Muhammad et al., 2020). As a result of this decreased traffic and transportation, there was a short-term decline in air pollutants such as NO_2. NO_2 is mainly a byproduct of the combustion of fossil fuels and the exhaust of vehicles. Besides polluting the atmosphere and posing a threat to human health, NO_2 is linked to eutrophication in coastal waters, smog, and acid rain (Wang & Su, 2020). Following the implementation of restricting public health policies around the world, NO_2 emissions declined by up to 30 percent in regions within China, Italy, France, Spain, and the United States (Muhammad et al., 2020). Declines in NO_2 were also observed and recorded by Dantas et al. (2020), the European Environment Agency (2020), Helm (2020), Kerimray et al. (2020), Lokhandwala and Gautam (2020), Wang and Su (2020), and Zambrano-Monserrate et al. (2020). In regions around the world, declines in other air pollutants such as $PM_{2.5}$, PM_{10}, CO, and SO_2 were also observed, though estimates were less consistent (Dantas et al., 2020; Hamway, 2020; Kerimray et al., 2020; Lokhandwala and Gautam, 2020; Wang & Su, 2020; Zambrano-Monserrate et al., 2020). These additional criteria air pollutants are also proven to cause disparate impacts to human health and the environment.

Yet while concentrations of these other air pollutants declined as first-order effects of public health policies, ground-level O_3 levels began to increase under lockdown policies as a second-order effect. Increases in O_3 were noted by (Arora et al., 2020; Kerimray et al., 2020; and Siciliano et al., 2020). This is due to the complex relationship on which ground-level ozone formation depends: O_3 forms when NO_x and volatile organic compounds (VOCs) react in the atmosphere in the presence of sunlight. Formation is dependent on the VOC/NO_x ratio in the atmosphere such that a reduction in NO_x will increase O_3 formation (Sicard et al., 2020). Since NO_2 decreased in numerous regions, it can be logically concluded that it contributed to an increase in ground-level ozone. This is a second-order environmental effect due to the fact that the change in ozone levels is partially dependent on the changes in concentration of other traffic-related air pollutants.

3.3.6 *Global Warming*

One of the main effects of the public health response to COVID-19 was the short-term reduction in global CO_2 levels, one of the primary greenhouse gases responsible for global warming. During the peak of the lockdown and travel restrictions in April 2020, daily global CO_2 emissions decreased by 17 percent. As discussed above, emissions fell in every sector except for residential emissions. Notable first-order reductions occurred in the power, aviation, surface transport, public, and industry sectors (Le Quéré et al., 2020a). In China, during the lockdown that included the Spring Festival Holiday, CO_2 emissions declined by about 25 percent (Wang & Su, 2020). This environmental effect was a direct first-order result of public health policies aimed at limiting the movement and interaction of people.

Short-term reductions in greenhouse gases were also observed as rippling second-order effects of restricting public health policies. Greenhouse gas emissions at the height of the lockdown period fell by 7.4 percent in the power sector, which accounts for energy conversion for electricity and heat generation. This was not only a first-order but a second-order effect of lockdown and travel restrictions due to the fact that power usage is distributed across all aspects of society. For example, changes in power usage at businesses may have decreased as a first-order effect while changes in power usage at a waste facility due to changes in the waste stream under COVID-19 could have been a second-order effect. Beyond this, emissions in the industry sector declined by 19 percent. In addition to being a first-order effect due to the direct decline of manpower available to drive industry, this is a second-order effect due to rippling impacts on economic productivity and trade. Furthermore, lockdown policies and economic decline led to a decline in global oil demand (Muhammad et al., 2020). Because the burning of oil and other fossil fuels are a critical source of anthropogenic greenhouse gas emissions, this is consistent with the above observations that greenhouse gas emissions declined, thereby positively affecting the global warming category.

3.3.7 *Environmental Degradation*

This category concerns harm to natural ecosystems, wildlife, and undeveloped or protected lands. A notable first-order effect that emerged during the height of the lockdown periods was a temporary reduction in noise pollution, particularly near major urban centers. Noise is sound that can cause a disturbance in communication, and it can interfere with sleep or the ability to concentrate. Environmental noise is unwanted sound that could be generated by anthropogenic activities (Zambrano-Monserrate et al., 2020). Noise from vehicles is one of the most significant contributors to noise pollution (Arora et al., 2020). Due to public health lockdowns and the reduction of vehicle usage and transport, noise pollution decreased (Arora et al, 2020; Zambrano-Monserrate et al., 2020). This likely had beneficial effects on natural ecosystems and wildlife located near urban centers.

The increased use of disinfectant in public spaces is also documented to show increased risks to urban wildlife. In response to COVID-19, widespread public disinfecting practices have become commonplace, with sanitation workers deployed to spray disinfectant in urban areas. This poses a risk to local wildlife due to the fact that many disinfectants include toxic chemicals such as chlorine and many of these species are inadvertently consuming these substances. This not only kills animals, but can also lead to the bioaccumulation of toxins within the food chain, spreading the toxins throughout an ecosystem. In February of 2020, hundreds of birds belonging to 17 different species died due to the widespread public usage of disinfectant in Chongqing, China (Nabi et al., 2020). This is a direct result of efforts undertaken to protect public health during the beginning of the coronavirus outbreak.

Another first-order effect of reduced human activity due to public health policies was in one instance a reduction in forest fires due to human activity. In Nepal, regions with smaller areas of community-managed forests per capita experienced an 8 percent reduction in the number of forest fires observed during its lockdown period. Overall, there was a negative correlation with forest fire incidents, indicating that the decline in human activity led to reduced environmental harm (Paudel, 2020). In other areas of the world such as the western coast of the United States, this trend was not reciprocated due to numerous climate- and weather-related factors.

With the greater usage of PPE and masks as a crucial part of the public health response to COVID-19, increased waste has led to greater instances of waste mismanagement. With greater numbers of individuals wearing masks as a personal precaution, there have been increased instances of individuals disposing of them in a way that is detrimental to the environment. Around the world, there is anecdotal evidence of discarded PPE washing up on beaches and in other natural places (Silva et al., 2020; Winters, 2020). This directly relates to Ring 2 as well due to the fact that PPE is being used as a part of both the medical response and public health response. As discussed in Ring 2, these single-use plastics take a long time to degrade and exist in the environment as microplastics for hundreds of years, posing a critical risk to the health of wildlife and polluting undisturbed natural areas (Prata et al., 2020). Because this aspect of the medical response is largely encompassed by the greater public health response, this effect is classified in this impact stage and environmental impact category rather than Ring 2.

A last first-order effect that has emerged within the literature relates to wildlife trade bans and changes to biodiversity protection. Following the proliferation of COVID-19 across the globe, scrutiny mounted for illegal wildlife trading and wild animal markets in countries such as China. In response to the SARS-CoV-2 outbreak, China announced the permanent ban of wildlife trading with the exception of trading for medicinal purposes (Gorman, 2020). Because wildlife trading is detrimental to biodiversity and conservation efforts, crackdowns on illegal trading may help protect natural wildlife populations and promote healthy ecosystems (UNODC, 2020). Therefore, changes to trading policies as a public health protection measure could help prevent further environmental degradation.

Most of the second-order effects stemming from the public health response to COVID-19 occurred as a result of lockdown policies and travel restrictions keeping individuals at home. One critical effect was the initial reduction in environmental monitoring. At the beginning of the pandemic, lockdown restrictions kept environmental protection officers and staff working at national parks and conservation areas home. This left many protected areas unmonitored and vulnerable to a rise in illegal deforestation, wildlife crime, poaching, and pollution (Hamwey, 2020; Helm, 2020). In general, risks to conservation and environmental protection efforts at this time were high. The other main second-order effect was a decline in ecotourism due to travel and lockdown restrictions. Ecotourism is a crucial industry for many countries because it benefits the economy while also providing funding for local environmental conservation and protection (Hamwey, 2020). Because of the decline in ecotourism activity and public health restrictions, natural areas were left vulnerable and unmonitored.

3.3.8 Summary

Overall, numerous environmental impacts have been observed due to various public health policies and measures implemented during the COVID-19 pandemic. Policies implemented around the world have included travel bans, lockdown and stay-at-home orders, social distancing measures, and mask mandates. Other initiatives have included public disinfecting practices and limitations on wildlife trafficking. At the same time, vaccinations were also developed in order to reduce transmission of the disease and prevent future outbreaks. These policies, initiatives, and decisions have led and will continue to lead to pronounced and dramatic effects on the natural environment as long as they are employed.

In regard to water pollution, reduced human recreation and industrial activity resulted in improved water quality and lower pollution levels in certain bodies of water. Public disinfecting practices, however, have likely led to a certain amount of water contamination. Changes have also occurred in relation to solid waste production. Policies such as the postponement of recycling programs, community waste sorting programs, and disposable bag bans influenced plastic waste streams. These waste streams have also been influenced by increased plastic demand due to the emphasis on masks and disposability as essential to sanitation. In addition, municipal and household waste streams were influenced by lockdown restrictions placed on populations—in some areas, municipal solid waste declined while household waste trends also demonstrated changes in both organic and inorganic waste production. Restrictions on travel also affected the agricultural and fishery export industries, with supplies suddenly unable to be shipped left to rot. Lastly, as vaccine campaigns have begun to be implemented, this will lead to greater levels of medical waste, and there is concern about the improper disposal of used syringes and other materials in the natural environment.

Beyond this, some of the most significant changes resulting from lockdown policies and travel restrictions were the changes observed in relation to air pollution and global warming factors. Following the implementation of these policies, which heavily restricted human movement, many regions saw a short-term improvement in air quality due to the reduction of air pollutant concentrations with less vehicles on the roads. The decline in transport mobility led to reductions in NO_2, $PM_{2.5}$, PM_{10}, CO, and SO_2 in numerous regions around the world, although there were also simultaneous observations of increases in ground-level O_3 due to chemical changes occurring within the atmosphere. This occurred at the same time that declines were observed in greenhouse gases responsible for global warming—numerous studies cited short-term declines in CO_2 during initial lockdown periods.

The general depression of human activity also led to notable impacts in the category of environmental degradation, with benefits including observed decreases in noise pollution levels, declines in human-induced forest fires in one area of the world, and greater efforts made to ban wildlife trafficking. Certain aspects of degradation occurred as well, with anecdotal evidence of increased PPE waste showing up in wild areas, public disinfection practices harming wildlife, and a reduction of manpower leading to reduced environmental monitoring and ecotourism.

Ring 3 is the most highly-populated ring out of the entire framework, with effects so extensive that it required the addition of a mechanism to differentiate between first- and second-order effects. The policies aimed at preventing transmission of the virus by preventing contact amongst people ultimately led to impacts (such as reductions in air pollution, water pollution, and greenhouse gas emissions) that were out of the realm of possibility prior to the emergence of SARS-CoV-2. As a result, it is clear that the public health policies implemented in response to the COVID-19 pandemic played a crucial role revealing many of the impacts that a human health crisis can have on the environment.

3.4   Ring 4: Effects of Adaptation and Rebound

3.4.1   *Introduction*

This ring discusses possible environmental effects that are stemming from the adaptation and eventual rebound of society during and after the COVID-19 pandemic. First, it is important to clarify that now that SARS-CoV-2 has spread to the extent that it has and has circulated in society for a significant period of time, causing severe reoccurrences in countries that once considered it under control, it is likely that it will never fully cease to exist in our society (Varlik, 2020). The only disease that has been fully eradicated through vaccination is smallpox, while others such as malaria, tuberculosis, and measles still exist and occur. There is currently indication that while COVID-19 as a pandemic will subside, it may still become endemic to society instead, with lower numbers of sustained transmission in the background of daily life (Varlik, 2020).

As the pandemic has wound on, countries and municipalities have spent considerable time developing protocols and procedures for adapting to the pandemic while trying to revitalize their economies. This has included policies geared towards allowing people back into public spaces while maintaining social distancing. As the influx of the initial first wave of cases started to subside, some governments were quick to start loosening lockdown restrictions and some travel restrictions, which resulted in increases in human activity that played a role in reversing many of the beneficial environmental effects observed in Ring 3. This has had an effect on all environmental impact categories and is discussed in depth below.

Throughout 2020, there was a global race to develop a vaccine as a crucial public health measure to SARS-CoV-2. There are also questions as to whether herd immunity will eventually develop as increasing numbers of individuals contract the virus, but this remains to be seen as medical experts do not know how long immunity to COVID-19 lasts after an individual has contracted it (Iwasaki, 2020; Kuebelbeck Paulsen, 2020). Furthermore, there is speculation among the community about whether COVID-19 could become seasonal, much like the influenza, which requires a vaccine every year to help prevent against different virus strains (Audi et al., 2020). While uncertainties remain, the COVID-19 pandemic is currently expected to subside slowly as vaccines are increasingly distributed. As the world returns to its "new normal," pronounced environmental effects might emerge as certain public health measures continue to be lifted. The full extent of these effects is not yet known. However, how the world responds will play a fundamental role in the effects that may be seen. This will come jointly from the large-scale actions and decisions made by public entities such as governments and businesses, but it will also come from personal, smaller-scale decisions made by individuals as consumers.

3.4.2   Large-Scale Rebound Effects

As discussed in Ring 3, unprecedented lockdown and travel restriction policies in 2020 led to a decline in economic output and an economic recession. As the world adapted to and eventually rebounds out of the pandemic, it will consequently try to rebound out of economic decline as businesses attempt to recover and continue increasing their profits. There is indication that as a result, most emissions declines seen during the pandemic due to reduced economic activity, shipping, and trade (discussed in Ring 3) will become fully reversed. Following the 2008 financial crisis, CO_2 emissions went through a rapid increase as the economy rebounded (Cheval, 2020). Though the recession that began occurring in 2020 has pronounced differences in comparison to the Great Recession, it is clear that if serious efforts are not made to continue curbing global emissions and making policy decisions that will effectively address climate change, any short-term reductions in emissions and pollution will be negligent as industry and trade ramp back up.

Even though the world has not fully rebounded from COVID-19 as the fall of 2020 brought a renewed surge in cases and a renewal of lockdowns worldwide, this revamp was already being observed over the summer as governments began loosening public health restrictions. In June 2020, news outlets reported a rebound in CO_2 emissions. While researchers found that there had been a 17 percent decline in CO_2 at the peak of lockdown efforts in early April of 2020 compared to the previous year, supplemental data found that this reduction had declined to only 4.7 percent by June. With the same industries, cars, and other pollutant-emitting facilities that existed before the pandemic, there was a high likelihood that emissions would return as "normal" activity levels resumed unless concerted efforts to create structural change were adopted. (Plumer & Popovich, 2020; Le Quéré et al., 2020b).

3.4.3   *Individual Activities and Their Effects*

This emissions reversal can also likely be attributed to individual activities beginning to go back to normal over the summer as certain restrictions were lifted. For example, transportation levels have rebounded in many countries since their original lockdown periods. According the Apple Inc.'s mobility data, many countries, including the United States, England, Canada, Italy, Germany, and other European countries, originally observed a steep drop in all forms of transportation during the peak of lockdown restrictions in March and April. By July and August, however, the data showed a gradual increase in the volume of people driving until it reached the same levels from before the pandemic or higher *(COVID-19 Mobility Trends Reports*, 2020). But as the pandemic worsened into the winter, with many countries reimplementing restrictions, driving levels in some regions declined again. In countries such as Japan, which was lauded for its quick and effective response to dealing with COVID-19 cases, driving and public transportation levels quickly rebounded and have remained high since (*COVID-19 Mobility Trends Reports*, 2020). Clearly, vehicle usage in many countries tracks closely with individual mobility, which has been controlled by government-imposed travel restrictions. As a result, it can be expected that transportation and its associated emissions will increase again following the full removal of pandemic travel restrictions.

Beyond driving and other day-to-day forms of transportation, it is worth exploring how air travel has responded with adaptation and will continue to respond with a gradual rebound. At this point, indication that air travel will increase is high as people are likely going to want to travel and go on vacation after being subjected to travel and lockdown restrictions of some capacity for a prolonged period of time. In October of 2020, the Transportation Security Administration (TSA) in the U.S. screened 1 million people in one day, marking the first time the administration's daily traveler count had reached that number since March (Schaper, 2020). Since peak lockdown periods, the TSA has reported a gradual increase in traveling numbers, indicating that there is a pent-up demand for air travel. Despite this, however, the number of air travelers was still reported to be down by 60 percent in comparison to the same time last year (Schaper, 2020). This, along with public transportation trends in certain countries may be indicative of long-term public distrust in public transportation, a subject which is discussed further in Ring 5.

There is also indication that the convenience of online shopping may cause this form of consumption to continue increasing even as society rebounds from COVID-19. Amazon.com, Inc. saw increased site traffic over the summer in July, with traffic up 28.1 percent compared to February even as coronavirus restrictions throughout the United States were being relaxed. This was an increase of nearly 9 percent when compared to the same month in 2019 (Ali, 2020). If this trend continues, the increase in plastic usage from the packaging of online shopping will most likely continue as demand remains high.

3.4.4   *Reversal of Effects from Ring 3*

Through the combined large-scale rebounding activities of governments, businesses, and industries and the individual-scale rebounding activities of the general public as consumers, many of the quantifiable environmental pollution reductions explored in Ring 3 will be reversed, at least to an extent. As discussed, emissions reductions are already declining, and it is likely that as society continues to rebound, this will get worse. The decline in greenhouse gas emissions also indicates that as industrial activities and transportation resume post-pandemic, air pollution will get worse again with NO_2, $PM_{2.5}$, PM_{10}, CO, and SO_2 levels likely to rise. Water pollution and noise pollution will likely increase again as well.

While waste trends are difficult to quantify in relation to the pandemic due to the fact that many different factors affect waste streams, a rebound of industrial and individual activities will likely lead to some reversals in waste trends observed under the pandemic. For example, municipal waste trends declined in many cities as people stayed home, accumulating their waste at home rather than in public spaces. As restrictions lift after the pandemic, however, and there is a return to the service economy as people dine out and occupy public spaces, municipal solid waste levels are likely going to increase back to at least pre-pandemic levels. With this return to the service economy, there may also be a decline in the amount of single-use plastic being used as take-out service declines and people are able to dine-in and use reusable dining materials and utensils. At the same time, due to possible long-term behavior changes, individuals may still prefer disposable plastic products in greater quantities if sanitation continues to be associated with disposability and people remain on edge about the transmission of viruses even after the pandemic subsides.

In regard to environmental degradation, with the lifting of certain lockdown restrictions and the encouragement of social distancing policies, many people were eager to reoccupy public spaces. In the United States, there has been an influx of visitors to national parks as states have slowly begun reopening, likely due to the fact that people want to get out of their houses safely and experience nature after being required to remain at home during unprecedented periods of lockdown. In the US, some parks began hitting capacity after opening back up during the pandemic, with rangers having to implement timed-entry policies. Unfortunately, however, this has led to an increase in environmental degradation as visitors have descended on these natural areas. Observations have included an increase in waste in various parks and graffiti or other forms of vandalism on trails (Chow, 2020). Furthermore, increased numbers of uninformed visitors are putting indigenous reservations (many of which are located in close proximity to national parks) at risk. Indigenous people in the United States are already disproportionately at risk from the pandemic due to their existing limited health services, weaker infrastructure, and higher rates of immunodeficiency diseases (Chow, 2020). As the original keepers of American land and the environment, this issue poses a unique environmental justice angle.

Beyond this, wildlife and ecosystem monitoring will likely go back to normal in many countries after the pandemic ends. With expected increases in travel, ecotourism will likely resurge from the decline experienced in the beginning of the year, aside from companies and industries that may have experienced permanent damage. This will lead to an increase in revenue flows for these industries, which will help support and encourage protection and maintenance of environmental areas. Waste and PPE in the environment, however, will probably continue due to the fact that we have not improved the way we dispose of and handle waste during the pandemic and due to the fact that people will likely continue to wear masks in many countries as a precaution long after the pandemic ends. Noise pollution is also expected to increase again as activities resume.

3.4.5 *Summary*

Ring 4 (adaptation and rebound) is one of the more fluid impact stages of this study's categorical framework. Over the course of 2020, adaptation unfolded as a slow process, with governments attempting to begin easing lockdown restrictions without allowing a massive rise in case numbers. Overtime, certain businesses were allowed to begin resuming operations, and life adjusted to the constantly-shifting new normal. One of the most notable changes observed during this period was the large-scale rebound effect of greenhouse gas emissions. Significant emissions declines observed in April of 2020 had receded by June, and experts were warning that greater action and sustainable societal change would be needed to maintain the necessary long-term decline required to prevent global warming from continuing to worsen.

Beyond the global level, however, trends in individual activities have changed as well as countries have adapted to the pandemic. As discussed, mobility trends in vehicle usage rebounded in many regions, which can be assumed to have led to rebounds in air pollutant concentrations. In some instances, air travel and public transportation have rebounded to a certain extent, which is also leading to an increase in air pollution and greenhouse gas emissions. In comparison to driving, these more public forms of transportation have been slower to recover, indicating a possibility for long-term trends to prevail.

It is the combination of both large-scale activity rebounds and individual activity choices that are contributing to the reversal of many of the environmental impacts observed in Ring 3. Preliminary observations indicate that improvements made in relation to air pollution, greenhouse gas emissions, and water pollution were likely reversed in many scenarios. Because of lightened lockdown policies, trends related to plastic waste streams are additionally expected to change due to the increase in people in public spaces. Other trends may continue despite the loosening of restrictions, such as sustained high levels of online commercial shopping (which can lead to greater consumption of plastic packaging). Overall, waste trends in general are expected to keep shifting as policies continue to affect the movement of people. However, due to the fact that there are a multitude of different factors at play and this research is not meant to be comprehensive, this section does not explore these possibilities. Assessing how certain waste trends, such as municipal waste trends, are expected to change is an opportunity for further research.

With increased human activity under adaptation and rebound, environmental degradation trends have also shifted. As countries such as the United States continued to adapt to the pandemic and slowly reopened national parks, a spike in visitation at many sites was observed, as well as increased levels of trash, pollution, and graffiti. Observations of PPE waste in the environment were expected to continue due to the prolonged wearing of masks under mask mandates and public health guidelines. At the same time, the return of greater environmental monitoring and ecotourism in some locations was expected to bolster the protection for natural lands that was missing during the initial lockdown and increase revenue for the conservation of natural areas.

Overall, findings for this ring were limited due to the fact that it was completed as adaptation to the pandemic began to occur. Numerous assumptions had to be made based on logical reasoning, and for this reason, Ring 4's population can be considered incomplete in this chapter.

3.5 Ring 5: Long-Term Effects

3.5.1 Introduction

Given the fact that the COVID-19 pandemic is ongoing, it is incredibly difficult to project the possible long-term environmental effects resulting from the pandemic and the way society rebounds out of it once it is over. In Ring 4, some of the possible activities that can be expected are discussed. In general, the trends in these activities and decisions will likely set us on one of two to three possible paths in the long run.

Some policy experts believe that greater government action during the coronavirus pandemic will lead to greater climate action as the world recovers, with greater investments in technology, science, and renewable energy sources centered at the heart of economic stimulus plans. Others, however, believe that emissions and pollution reductions will be solely short-term, leading to minimal net reductions for the year, and that climate policies will face a political setback as they are postponed in favor of rapid industrial recovery with traditional energy sources (Pearce, 2020).

Gillingham et al. (2020) presents more of an economist's view of these two options: If the pandemic ends sooner rather than later and the economy rebounds quickly, long-term effects will be minimal. However, it the pandemic persists and causes a significant global recession, there will be negative long-run consequences for the success and adoption of clean energy technologies. It is, however, important to note that if the pandemic ends sooner, other polluting industries will experience fewer long-term effects as well, not just renewable industries. This is a subject that must be further explored.

Cheval et al. (2020) presents three paths for how the world could respond to the COVID-19 pandemic, including: (1) There is a widescale change in behavior and a regime shift due to the shock of the pandemic and its consequences, (2) the world goes back to the old normal, in which affairs are carried out "business-as-usual," and (3) the world goes beyond "back to normal" and rebounds even more aggressively, with adverse impacts for people and the environment. While the first is optimistic, the latter two are pessimistic.

Based on the rebounding emissions statistics discussed in Ring 4, there is indication that we may be already set on following one of the latter two negative rebound paths. This will likely occur as governments and businesses continue to prioritize a quick economic recovery over a sustainable recovery. While economic recovery is important, experts have stressed the fact that this should not continue to come at the expense of the climate. Beyond just the wellbeing of the planet and its ecosystems, however, there are further public health considerations to keep in mind—cleaner air and water help protect against the spread of diseases, which is only getting worse with the rapid globalization society has witnessed in the past century alone. For example, it was found that higher air pollution in communities has correlated with greater susceptibility to COVID-19 (Fattorini & Regoli, 2020). In considering how to prevent future pandemics and the economic decline that they can bring, governments may look to consider the fact that environmental pollution only worsens public health.

3.5.2 *Changes in Domestic and International Policy and Cooperation*

Beyond examining different recovery paths, experts are also exploring the possibility of more specific long-term consequences. One area that may be impacted is that of policy changes and international cooperation in environmental agreements. If the current economic decline persists, there is a chance that climate change mitigation targets and policies could either be delayed, relaxed, or scrapped altogether as governments shift their focus to prioritizing economic rebound and recovery over long-term climate protection (Gillingham et al., 2020; Helm, 2020).

3.5.3 *Changes in Transportation*

The future of public transportation is also in question given the reverberating effects that the COVID-19 pandemic may have on society. With the decline in transport and mobility discussed in Rings 3 and 4, there are possible implications for the future of public transportation, even after the pandemic is considered over. Mobility trends in certain countries such as the United States and Canada have shown that despite driving trends slowly rebounding after the steep drop in all forms of transportation in March and April, use of public transportation has remained low. In the US, national transit ridership fell nearly 10 percent in the first quarter of 2020 compared to 2019, dropping by over 40 percent in March (Olin, 2020). Experts are finding that ridership is not rebounding at the speed that driving has, indicating a possible shift for the future of transportation trends. As public transportation is an important factor in keeping polluting vehicles off of the roads, this would negatively impact the process of trying to reduce greenhouse gas emissions. This also has implications for the nature of life in cities, where higher numbers of people driving cars can lead to greater congestion and air pollution.

3.5.4 *Changes in Urban Geography*

A localized long-term trend being witnessed is a change in city life due to the movement of people out of cities and into the suburbs. In cities, where an estimated 55 percent of the world's population is located and where coronavirus has hit the hardest, there is the possibility that the very fabric of life could change for the long-term (United Nations Department of Economic and Social Affairs, 2018). While most are in consensus about the fact that COVID-19 will by no means destroy the existence of cities, there is still discussion of many of the changes that could occur within these urban centers. Some experts have acknowledged that the fear of human density on public transportation and in day-to-day life may push wealthier families to move towards the suburbs (Florida et al., 2020). This trend has been debated due to the fact that even though moving numbers were down across the country as a result of stay-at-home orders and travel restrictions, certain American cities such as San Francisco and New York City have witnessed significant changes in moving patterns, with more individuals leaving these cities than moving into them from mid-March to the end of June in 2020 (Patino, 2020). In New York, many city residents are reportedly moving to the suburbs, with suburban real estate agents attesting to higher numbers of inquiries and offers for suburban properties in the greater New York City area (Berliner, 2020). It is clear that these trends are very localized, however, so there is no indication yet that this will become a pronounced long-term trend. In addition, the ability to move during a pandemic is likely afforded only by wealthier members of society, therefore making this trend separate from reality for many.

Many also see long-term possibilities for a change in the way we build back our cities, with planners now having the chance to implement changes that promote smarter density of public spaces and greener infrastructure. This is seen as a chance to kick-start greater implementation of circular economics, climate-resilient structures, and greater equality (Florida et al., 2020). Should these changes occur, this will benefit not only people but the natural environment.

3.5.5 *Changes in Economy and Business*

Other experts are noting that the shift to digital retail, a cashless economy, remote work, and other virtual services are changing the way city dwellers live (Florida et al., 2020). As discussed in Ring 4, sustained preference for online retail and home delivery for many different types of goods could lead to long-term trends in greater plastic waste generation due to the packaging associated with the shipping and transport of goods. With greater parts of city life shifting online, less commuting may cause fewer emissions and pollution, while residential emissions could increase from greater numbers of people staying home. Greater dependence and utilization of the internet by more parts of public life could lead to greater energy usage overall.

As the pandemic has continued, there has also been a shift in how many forms of business are being conducted that will likely pervade long after it has ended. Two main changes that have occurred have been the shift to remote work and the greater utilization of online services (Brynjolfsson et al., 2020). Businesses may also downsize in order to lower office costs, staggering between shifts of workers entering the office and working at home. This may lead to changes in waste and emissions trends associated with the business sector, keeping workplace energy usage and solid waste production lower than pre-pandemic levels. Other changes in emissions from this remain to be explored—with greater numbers of employees working from home, residential emissions and household waste will likely increase. International conferences that once had individuals traveling across the globe could become conducted virtually across the board, with members tuning in from their homes around the world instead. This could have important ramifications for emissions from the aviation sector.

3.5.6 *Changes in Behavior*

Overall, many of these changes will stem from general shifts in human behavior following the pandemic. As discussed, the continued widespread fear of germs could lead to a prolonged decline in ridership of public transit. This would inhibit the good that these transportation methods do for urban greenhouse gas emissions. There is also the possibility that health fears could lead to greater general levels of mask-wearing as a precaution around the world. Whereas numerous Asian countries such as South Korea, China, and Japan have long normalized the public wearing of face masks, greater adopted usage over the long-term could have a more pronounced effect of PPE on the waste stream through greater plastic generation and usage. Lastly, this fear could lead to the sustained preference of disposable goods over reusable goods due to the widespread perpetuation of the myth that sanitation comes with disposability. This would negatively impact waste generation.

This also ties into the fact that the social life of cities will change as people may continue to prefer staying in over going out into public spaces. As discussed above and in Ring 4, with greater numbers of people staying home and ordering the things they need online, waste from disposable packaging is extremely likely to remain higher than it used to be.

There is also the argument that the COVID-19 pandemic has led to a major change in information through its proliferation in the news and on social media, creating a shared experience for a large number of people that may shift how many make choices (Helm, 2020). The negative shocks of the entire ordeal could make people more averse to risks and more likely to save more, which could reduce the willingness to pay for benefits to the environment (Helm, 2020). At the same time, however, environmental spaces, especially in urban areas, could become more highly valued. An increased appreciation for the environment could emerge after the respite that it has brought so many during these long months of stay-at-home orders, reduced activities, and a general limit on what one would consider "normal life." As discussed in Ring 3, greater numbers of people who had access to the outdoors were getting outside during the months of quarantine—a fact demonstrated by the greater amount of degradation and trash found on nature paths and in natural parks.

Helm also discusses whether the experience of the coronavirus could make people shift towards collectivism or individualism. Greater collectivism would favor greater international cooperation over climate policies aimed at solving the climate crisis. Individualism, which would stem from a greater tendency to prefer social isolation, would likely favor less cooperation. Of course, many other factors influence these types of mindsets, especially in a world with incredibly diverse countries that have their own respective histories, cultures, and priorities. In the future, however, these changes in psychological behavior in relation to COVID-19 are worth exploring.

*3.5.7 **Summary***

Because the COVID-19 pandemic has influenced almost every aspect of life, there are distinct possibilities for long-term trends that may prevail long after the pandemic is considered to be over. Some of these possibilities includes changes in the way domestic and international communities view climate change—because economic stability is often valued ahead of environmental vitality, future policies regarding emissions targets and other climate commitments on the international stage may be weakened or pushed to the side.

Long-term trends may also be observed in public transportation. The lack of rebound in public transit ridership may be indicative of a long-term consumer preference for driving, which could seriously affect greenhouse gas emissions and air pollution levels in urban areas. Urban geography is another realm in which long-term changes may occur due to urban flight to the suburbs during the pandemic. At the same time, opportunities are emerging to improve urban spaces and make them more climate-resilient, healthy, and equitable moving forward.

Beyond this, some are predicting long-term changes in how our economy functions and how business is conducted. Shifts to greater digital retail, a cashless economy, remote work, and other virtual services have already transformed workspaces and businesses as society continued to find ways to function and connect under lockdown restrictions and other policies that prevented human contact. These changes have major implications for waste, emissions, energy usage, air pollution, and other environmental indicators, especially due to the fact that large scale changes like these will impact nearly every aspect of human life.

In the end, many of these changes will occur due to long-term shifts in human behavior and preferences. The fear of germs and the preference for more space and cleaner air may contribute to the long-term trends in transportation, urban geography, and economy and business discussed above. All of these will have differing impacts on the environment, but because these possibilities are so abstract, Ring 5 is not sub-divided into the environmental impact categories presented by this paper. While most impacts discussed in this section have not been thoroughly explored within the literature due to the unprecedented magnitude of COVID-19's medical and public health policies and their subsequent effects, they have implications for understanding some of the long-term effects that a public health crisis can have on the environment. For this reason, further research is required in the future to adequately understand these effects.

3.6 Summary and Framework Population

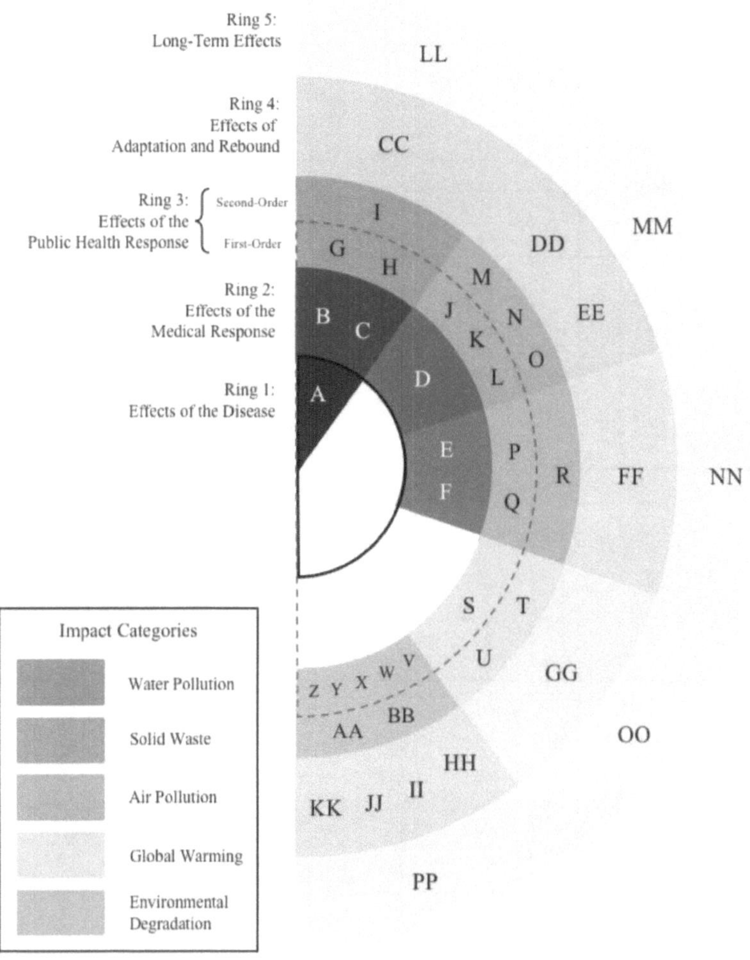

Figure 2. Observed and Expected Environmental Impacts of the COVID-19 Pandemic. The framework has been populated through a review of emerging literature on the environmental effects of the COVID-19 pandemic and existing literature on environmental impacts of the health care sector. See Table 1 for corresponding effect descriptions. Note: Figure is not comprehensive.

Table 1: Observed and Expected Environmental Impacts of the COVID-19 Pandemic

	Water Pollution	Solid Waste	Air Pollution	Global Warming	Environmental Degradation
Ring 1: **Effects of the Health Issue**	A. Confirmed cases of the presence of the virus in wastewater systems, which could be another source of transmission	No observed effects	No observed effects	No observed effects	No observed effects
Ring 2: **Effects of the Medical Response**	B. Probable increase in pollution from antiviral usage C. Probable increase in pollution from disinfectant usage	D. Increase in medical waste from the treatment of more patients	E. Increased air pollution from medical waste incineration F. Increased air pollution from improper burning of medical waste	No observed effects outside of the existing impacts of the health care system	No observed effects outside of the existing impacts of the health care system
Ring 3: **First-Order Effects of the Public Health Response**	G. Decline in water pollution from reduction in recreational activity H. Probable increase in water pollution due to disinfectant usage in public spaces	J. Increase in plastic waste K. Changes in municipal solid waste and household waste trends L. Probable increase in medical waste due to eventual improper vaccine disposal	P. Short-term decline in NO_2 emissions from reduction in mobility Q. Short-term declines in other air pollutants such as $PM_{2.5}$, PM_{10}, CO, and SO_2 from reduction in mobility	S. Short-term decline in emissions of greenhouse gases such as CO_2	V. Decline in noise pollution W. Increase in harm to wildlife due to disinfectant use in public X. Decline in forest fires in certain areas of the world Y. Increase in environmental pollution from increased PPE waste Z. Increase in wildlife trade bans and biodiversity protection
Second-Order Effects of the Public Health Response	I. Decline in water pollution from reduction in industrial activity	M. Increase in plastic waste from disposable packaging N. Decrease in plastic demand in certain non-medical sectors O. Increase in organic waste from declines in fishery and other exports	R. Short-term increase in ground-level ozone pollution	T. Short-term decline in emissions of greenhouse gases such as CO_2 U. Short-term decline in global oil demand	AA. Decline in environmental monitoring and protection enforcement BB. Decline in ecotourism and associated environmental protection
Ring 4: **Effects of Adaptation and Rebound**	CC. Expected reversal in water pollution reductions from rebounded activity	DD. Possible changes in the usage of disposable plastic due to increase in dining in and sustained preference for disposable goods EE. Expected increase in municipal solid waste	FF. Expected reversal in air pollution reductions	GG. Expected reversal in short-term emissions declines	HH. Increase in degradation from greater national park patronage in certain places II. Expected improvement in environmental monitoring and ecotourism JJ. Continued waste and PPE pollution in the environment KK. Expected rebound in noise pollution levels
Ring 5: **Long-Term Effects**	LL. Changes in domestic and international policy and cooperation: Relaxed/delayed climate change mitigation targets MM. Changes in transportation: Long-term decline in usage of public transportation NN. Changes in behavior: Increase in plastic waste from higher usage of masks and preference for disposable goods OO. Changes in urban geography: Increase in movement to the suburbs, increase in building of green infrastructure and de-densification of public spaces PP. Changes in economy and business: Shift to digital/virtual services and economy leading to an increase in plastic waste generation; Decline in commuting-related emissions, increase in residential emissions, decline in workplace energy usage and waste production				

Addendum:
Additional notable and observed effects that fall under Ring 1 but cannot be adequately classified by existing impact categories:
- Increase in human mortality
- Cases of reverse zoonotic transmission

Table 1. Summary of Observed and Expected Environmental Impacts of the COVID-19 Pandemic.

48

Chapter 4: Case Study Application

4.1   Case Study #1: Severe Acute Respiratory Syndrome (SARS) Outbreak (2003)

4.1.1   Introduction

Severe acute respiratory syndrome (SARS) is a viral respiratory disease caused by a coronavirus called SARS-CoV (CDC, n.d.). The SARS outbreak originated in China in February of 2003 (WHO, n.d.). Following the outbreak, the disease spread to over two dozen countries in North America, South America, Europe, and Asia before its containment, and it is thought to have infected 8,098 individuals worldwide, killing 774 (CDC, n.d.). The illness is transmitted mainly by airborne respiratory droplets and through surfaces, and symptoms include a high fever, headache, body aches, and pneumonia. Other symptoms can include diarrhea and a dry cough (CDC, n.d.). A notable difference between COVID-19 and SARS are the diseases' mortality rates. At the time of the 2003 outbreak, SARS had a higher mortality rate of 9.7 percent, while current estimates for COVID-19 range from about 1-3.5 percent in some of the most affected countries (not including Mexico, which is an outlier at 8.7 percent) (Petersen et al., 2020; Johns Hopkins Coronavirus Resource Center [JHCRC], 2021). With regard to transmission, the R0 or reproduction number indicates how contagious a disease is, with a value over 1 indicating that an outbreak or epidemic is growing. The R0 of SARS-CoV can be estimated at about 2.4, while scientists are currently estimating the R0 of SARS-CoV-2 to be about 2.5 (with some estimates even higher) (Petersen et al., 2020). Though COVID-19 has been more transmissible than SARS was at the time of its outbreak, SARS had a higher mortality rate.

As discussed in Chapter 1, most research on the intersection of the environment and public health has historically focused on the role of environmental factors such as pollution in worsening public health issues. This is true in the case of the SARS outbreak as well, as a basic search on the SARS outbreak and the environment yields numerous studies on the role of air pollution and other factors in contributing to the spread of SARS. Coverage of SARS and the effects it may have had on the environment is sparse due to the fact that there was far less of a focus on environmental monitoring at the time than there is today. For this reason, employing the framework populated by COVID-19 helps serve as a guide in researching any environmental effects that may have occurred as a result of the SARS outbreak.

4.1.2   Ring 1: Effects of the Health Issue

4.1.2.1   Introduction

In implementing the framework developed in Chapter 3, it is necessary to examine the potential effects that the SARS outbreak had on people and the environment. This section explores two of the three effects observed from COVID-19: human mortality and water impacts. A review of existing literature yielded no findings on the possible impact of SARS on other species.

4.1.2.2   Water Impacts

In the aftermath of the SARS outbreak, there was indication that the disease could be spread through fecal-oral transmission from contaminated wastewater. Wang et al. (2005) found the RNA of SARS-CoV in the sewage of two hospitals before disinfection. While the samples were not infectious, the study suggested that SARS-CoV could be excreted through the stool or urine of patients into sewage, which made the sewage system a possible source of transmission for the disease. This possibility was also suggested by Peiris et al. (2003) and Tomlinson and Cockram (2003) in the case of a major outbreak in Hong Kong in which 321 people in a housing estate contracted the illness. SARS-CoV was also reported in stool samples by Chan et al. (2004) and Liu et al. (2004). Both suggested that excreted SARS-CoV may be less infectious. Gundy et al. (2008), noted this lack of consensus regarding the contagiousness of SARS-CoV in wastewater and argued for greater research into this possibility. This study concluded that in general, coronaviruses die off quickly in wastewater but that their survival is highly dependent on water temperature. Overall, there seems to be a lack of consensus on the ability of SARS-CoV to persist in sewage systems, but transmission via this route was suggested as the cause for one of the most severe localized outbreaks in the region at the time. As a result, the virus that causes SARS can be considered likely to impact water systems.

4.1.2.3   Human Mortality

As was discussed in Chapter 3, it is important to include the effect of SARS on human life due to its significance. Though only 8,098 individuals were infected worldwide, 774 died from the disease, giving the SARS outbreak of 2003 a fairly high mortality rate in comparison to COVID-19 (CDC, n.d.). In comparison to COVID-19, the SARS outbreak recorded far fewer deaths despite the fact that this disease had a higher mortality rate.

4.1.2.4 Summary

In general, documented direct impacts of SARS-CoV itself are limited due to the smaller-scale nature of the original outbreak. Though studies were performed on the possible persistence of SARS-CoV in wastewater systems and wastewater transmission was a suspected cause of one of the most intense local outbreaks of SARS, there is a lack of consensus on the full extent of the impacts that SARS-CoV viral loading may have had at the time. Because the outbreak ended relatively quickly and has since remined contained, little research has since focused on this topic. Impacts on human mortality were limited in comparison to the COVID-19 pandemic, with 774 deaths occurring due to the virus' lower transmission rate and precautions taken at the time.

4.1.3   Ring 2: Effects of the Medical Response

4.1.3.1 Introduction

As discussed in Chapter 3, Yang et al. (2020) classifies adequate response measures to a viral disease through the four following categories: rapid response, treatment, reducing viral transmission, and prevention. This paper divides these categories into two different but overlapping aspects of a response: the medical response and the public health response. Measures focusing on the rapid response, detection, and treatment all fall under the realm of the SARS medical response. A key part of authorities' rapid response to the SARS outbreak was testing, which was carried out through RNA tests, serologic tests, and viral culture analysis (Chan et al., 2004). In this case, reducing transmission overlaps with the public health response but applies to preventing transmission of SARS within health care facilities. To reduce viral spread during medical care and within society in general, Chinese public health officials implemented the isolation of SARS patients, quarantine of contacts, and the use of PPE by health care workers among other strategies (CDC, 2003). The standard treatment of SARS at the time of the outbreak in regions such as Hong Kong included the use of antivirals and corticosteroids, and disinfectant was used to sanitize health care facilities (Tai, 2007; Shaw, 2006). These various methods implemented as a part of the medical response in the worst areas of the SARS outbreak led to varying impacts on different environmental categories.

4.1.3.2 Water Pollution

While there is currently no vaccine available to prevent against SARS nor a specific antiviral treatment (due to the fact that SARS disappeared before major vaccine development could undergo enough testing), existing antivirals and corticosteroids were tested in treatment. Antiviral treatment included the use of drugs such as ribavirin and a combination of lopinavir and ritonavir (Chu et al., 2004; Tai, 2007). Aside from a lack of consensus over which treatment courses were effective, the use of these types of antivirals indicates that there was a potential for wastewater accumulation and ecotoxicity at this time. As discussed in Chapter 3, lopinavir, which is also being tested in treating COVID-19, has a high bioaccumulation potential in wastewater streams and could possibly pose an ecotoxicological risk (Race et al., 2020). ritonavir, on the other hand, is hydrophobic and tends to absorb onto suspended solids in aquatic systems, so it has low accumulation levels (Nannou et al., 2020). There is little information available on potential environmental effects of ribavirin.

During the 2003 SARS outbreak, there was a consensus among medical experts that the cleaning and disinfection of hospital surfaces using common disinfectants was effective against SARS-CoV, leading to the implementation of this practice in medical facilities (Shaw, 2006). As a result, it can be inferred that disinfectant may have ended up in water bodies due to drainage and sewage systems in hospitals and other medical facilities. As discussed in Chapter 3, common disinfectants, especially bleach, can end up reacting with other compounds in a water compartment, leading to the production of ecotoxic by-products that can be harmful to marine organisms (Zhang et al., 2020).

4.1.3.3 Solid Waste

The 2003 SARS outbreak contributed to higher levels of hospital waste during the height of the crisis, but leveled off fairly quickly in comparison to the elevated levels of waste that have been observed during the COVID-19 pandemic. This was in part due to the fact that health care workers were required to wear PPE such as gowns, gloves, N95 or higher respirators, and eye protection (McDonald et al., 2004). A study of one Taiwanese hospital during the 2003 SARS outbreak reported that the amount of infectious medical waste increased from 0.85 kg per patient-day to 2.7 kg per patient day at the height of the epidemic. The study found that waste generation returned to normal levels in only 10 days (Chiang et al., 2006). This study is indicative of the likely trend that medical waste increased at the time as a result of the health crisis.

4.1.3.4   Air Pollution

A review of the literature returned no specific articles regarding the incineration of waste during the SARS epidemic. A notable effect of the epidemic itself, however, was that it forced China to pay greater attention to the disposal and treatment of biomedical waste following the outbreak. At the time of the outbreak, incineration was not a common method of medical waste disposal. Instead, medical waste was often mixed with municipal solid waste, and steam sterilization treatment was only applied to highly infectious waste (Zhao et al., 2009). From this, it can be inferred that with the absence of heavy lockdown policies during the SARS outbreak, changes in air pollution stemming from the health crisis were minimal.

4.1.3.5   Summary

Overall, literature on direct documented impacts of the SARS medical response on the environment was limited. For this reason, logical reasoning was used to draw conclusions about the impacts that likely stemmed from antiviral and disinfectant use. The most significant finding from this section was the fact that infectious medical waste increased during the outbreak in Taiwan, an effect that likely occurred elsewhere in regions seriously affected by the disease. The fact that only one article in the literature reported on medical waste trends related to SARS is indicative of how analysis of environmental impacts from health crises at the time was considered far less of a priority than it is now. Regarding air pollution, this observation is also applicable—there was no clear information available on the air quality impacts of medical waste incineration due to the fact that incineration practices were not common in countries such as China in the early 2000s. In researching this impact category, however, it became apparent that the outbreak impacted the country's approach towards medical waste disposal moving forward, a trend that is discussed more in depth in Ring 5.

4.1.4   Ring 3: Effects of the Public Health Response

4.1.4.1   Introduction

Though SARS was first thought to have emerged in the Guangdong Province of China in late 2002, it wasn't fully acknowledged and dealt with through a full-scale public health response until March and April of 2003. With the virus spreading, news about it spread informally among the general public, eventually reaching the international health community (Institute of Medicine, 2004). Pressure mounted on the Chinese government to act, and the WHO issued its first global warning about SARS on March 12, followed by a groundbreaking travel advisory on March 15 (WHO, 2003a; WHO, 2003b). As the virus continued to spread to other countries such as Vietnam and Canada through air travel, the WHO took unprecedented steps in recommending the suspension of all but essential travel to SARS-affected areas, including Hong Kong, Beijing, Guangdong Province, and Shanxi Province in China and Toronto, Canada (WHO, 2003c). Throughout this time, the gravity of the SARS outbreak was continuously downplayed by Chinese health officials. By the end of April, however, amid growing public outcry, the national and local governments began to mobilize, removing officials for their role in mismanaging the crisis (Huang, 2004).

With this development, numerous public health measures were rapidly enforced. Villages, housing complexes, and other residential areas suspected of outbreaks were cut off, thousands of individuals were quarantined, and screening checkpoints were set up to monitor temperatures (Huang, 2004). In Beijing, it is estimated that approximately 30,000 people were subjected to quarantine (CDC, 2003). In addition to the isolation and quarantining of contacts, school and university education was paused, and district-wide disinfecting was occurring (Hung, 2003). Around the world, airports implemented public health notices to alert travelers as well as entry and exit temperature screening (Wilder-Smith, 2006). Surveillance of global communications, contact tracing, and quarantine were ultimately key to containing the virus and reducing transmission in countries around the world. By July, the WHO announced the effective end of the pandemic after it found that all chains of transmission had been broken (Institute of Medicine, 2004; Wilder-Smith, 2006).

4.1.4.2 Water Pollution

Because the widespread use of disinfectant was documented during both the medical and public health response to the SARS outbreak, it is reasonable to assume that there was a greater level of environmental pollution at this time. A particular concern with the use of disinfectants is the potential for water pollution due to runoff and the draining of sewage systems. In Hong Kong, the government reportedly released numerous public service announcements advising residents to thoroughly disinfect their homes with solutions of bleach and water in order to combat the spread of the virus (Lau et al., 2004). Chlorine disinfectants, once in natural water bodies, have the potential to chemically bond with other compounds in water, forming toxic by-products that can be harmful to marine plants and animals (Zhang et al., 2020). The assumptions made within this ring can be extended to understanding water impacts mentioned in Ring 2 as disinfectant was used in medical facilities as part of the medical response to SARS, which was closely intertwined with the public health response.

4.1.4.3 Solid Waste

A key part of the public health response to the SARS outbreak was the implementation of public health measures designed to increase social distancing. Aside from cancelling mass gatherings and closing schools and other public facilities, some high-risk areas chose to require masks for citizens who were using public transport, working in restaurants, or entering medical facilities (Bell, 2004). Mask wearing also became more common as people made the choice to wear one in public. While there is no direct data available regarding how widespread mask-wearing became, it can be assumed that the higher usage of PPE at this time likely lead to greater levels of plastic waste in local waste streams at the time.

4.1.4.4 Global Warming

The WHO's travel advisories combined with government-issued travel recommendations around the world contributed to a marked decrease in air travel to Asia and Canada. During the outbreak, global passenger traffic fell by 18.5 percent in April 2003 compared to the same period in 2002. The Asia Pacific region was hit particularly hard, with a decline of nearly 45 percent compared to the year before. Overall, passenger traffic did not return to normal for nine months (Pham, 2020). According to the International Air Transport Authority, the SARS outbreak cost Asia Pacific airlines $6 billion and North American airlines $1 billion (Pham, 2020). Though the SARS outbreak caused a depressed level of air travel however, there is no indication that aviation emissions declined at the time. This is likely due to the fact that aviation emissions have been steadily trending upward in the past 50 years as a result of continuously increasing passenger loads despite energy intensity improvements that have been made within the sector (Environmental and Energy Study Institute [EESI], 2019). If anything, the SARS outbreak may have played a role in contributing to a plateau in emissions before they continued their rapid increase in the years following. This is supported by He and Xu's (2012) estimation of China's aviation emissions from 1960-2009, which documented a minimal change in CO_2 levels between 2002 and 2003 before jumping up in 2004. This trend correlates with global aviation emissions, which continued to trend upward with passenger transport volumes despite events such as the World Trade Center attack in 2001 and the SARS outbreak in 2003 (Lee et al., 2009).

4.1.4.5   Regarding the Categories of Air Pollution and Environmental Degradation

As the outbreak of SARS was not severe enough to require extensive lockdown policies and border closings in the way that COVID-19 has, there is no documentable evidence of any direct or indirect environmental impacts on air pollution or environmental degradation stemming from the health crisis. There is a possibility, of course, that increased mask wearing and PPE usage could have led to greater environmental pollution, but there is no evidence that this was observed at the time. The only aspect of the public health response that may have temporarily impacted environmental degradation was the implementation of a temporary ban on the trade and consumption of wild animals at lower legislative levels of government due to the concern that the virus had originated from an animal (Koh et al., 2021). However, these were so short-lived that the effects of these policies on biodiversity conservation or endangered animal protection are not documented.

4.1.4.6   Summary

Overall, the public health measures implemented in areas most intensely affected by SARS were quite severe for the time period once government officials acted. Areas suspected of localized outbreaks were cut off and isolated, thousands were subject to contact tracing and quarantine, and numerous aspects of public life such as education were put on pause to lessen the transmission of the virus. Relating to the categories of water impacts and solid waste, most evidence of any impacts stems from anecdotal evidence and logical conclusions drawn from policy guidelines at the time. Because disinfection was widely used and promoted by governments at the time, it is reasonable to assume that these products made their way into local water systems. Numerous disinfecting agents can have varying effects on waterways and their ecological inhabitants. Regarding solid waste, some areas required the use of face masks to lower transmission for the sake of public health. It can be assumed that the greater overall use of PPE impacted the solid waste system at the time, but a lack of available data and the fact that the specifics of this are beyond the scope of this paper dismisses the potential to make any quantitative conclusions about these impacts.

Despite the public health measures taken, the SARS outbreak was not intense enough to provoke large-scale travel restrictions or national border closings. For this reason, most global warming impacts stemmed from human fear and behavioral changes. At the time of the outbreak, air passenger traffic declined especially in the Asia Pacific region, but this ultimately only contributed to a plateauing of aviation emissions in China. Furthermore, some of the larger-scale effects that were observed during the COVID-19 pandemic were not observed or studied during the SARS outbreak. Very limited information was available regarding the environmental impact categories of air pollution and environmental degradation. The only information related to possible environmental degradation impacts was a temporary ban on the trade and consumption of wild animals, but there is no indication that these policies had any effect on biodiversity conservation or endangered animal preservation.

4.1.5 Ring 4: Effects of Adaptation and Rebound

4.1.5.1 Introduction

Findings for environmental effects of the adaptation and rebound of society to SARS are sparse. This is most likely explained by the fact that the SARS outbreak was short-lived, only lasting a little over half of a year. In addition, since lockdown policies and public health measures weren't prolonged, there wasn't much of a depression in an activity to rebound from. As a result, conclusions in this impact stage cannot be made about the categories of water pollution, solid waste, or environmental degradation.

4.1.5.2 Air Pollution

Following the SARS outbreak, the Chinese government pushed stimulus efforts for economic recovery with the goal of offsetting the negative economic impacts of the crisis. This led to an "investment boom" and rebound in industry, which contributed to higher levels of particulate matter pollution in the region surrounding Beijing (Centre for Research on Energy and Clean Air [CREA], 2020). Aside from this article, a search of the literature yielded no other documentation regarding changes in air pollution levels in China or nearby regions at the time. Any further information may be available via local government agency websites.

4.1.5.3 Global Warming

There is a chance that changes in aviation during and after the SARS outbreak may have affected global warming. As discussed in Ring 3, unprecedented travel advisories issued by the WHO at the time led to a significant decline in global aviation levels, most notably in the Asia Pacific region. Despite these declines however, these trends only contributed to a plateau in aviation emissions at most. Following the end of the outbreak and the subsequent lifting of travel advisories, it is important to note that aviation ridership once again increased, leading to an increase in emissions compared to 2003 and the years before (He & Xu, 2012; Lee et al., 2009). This jump may have been due to the investment boom and rebound in industry spurred on by the Chinese government following the health crisis, as cited by CREA (2020). It also could have been due to the already increasing trends in emissions levels due to increasing passenger loads, globalization, and improvements in technology.

4.1.5.4 Summary

Generally, the application of Ring 4 to the SARS outbreak is highly limited due to the fact that the outbreak was relatively short-lived and did not require the population most seriously affected by the crisis to semi-permanently adapt to it. There was a lack of findings related to the impact categories of water pollution, solid waste, and environmental degradation, though these topics may benefit from further exploration. Conclusions made about air pollution are largely speculative due to reports of an investment boom and rebound of industry in China following the end of the outbreak, but one report within the literature mentions in increase in localized air pollution. The most significant finding falls within the category of global warming, as CO_2 emissions from global aviation continued to climb after plateauing during the SARS epidemic and other significant historical events such as the September 11th attack on the Twin Towers in New York City. Aviation emission quickly rebounded, spurred on by increasing passenger loads, increasing globalization and connectivity, and technological innovation. This is evidence of the fact that many large-scale environmental impacts that come from behavioral changes during a public health or geopolitical crisis are largely reversible.

4.1.6 Ring 5: Long-Term Effects

4.1.6.1 Introduction

The SARS outbreak represented a wake-up call for many governments due to its severity and potential for massive disruptions in public life. Particularly in China, which was one of the most heavily impacted nations during this time, the public failure to contain the outbreak and take it seriously as well as the general disorder caused by the virus itself caused a shift in the Chinese health care system moving forward. Numerous changes were made in order to modernize and improve the organization and structure of the health care system for the purpose of better responding to another health crisis like SARS should it happen again. Long-term changes were also made to the way solid medical waste was handled for disposal.

4.1.6.2 Changes in Management of Solid Medical Waste

As was briefly discussed in Ring 2, a notable effect of the SARS outbreak was that it forced China to devote greater attention and resources to the disposal and treatment of hazardous medical waste in the years following the crisis. At the time of the outbreak, incineration was not a common method of disposal. Medical waste was often mixed with municipal solid waste, and steam sterilization treatment was only applied to highly infectious waste. A large amount of dangerous infectious hospital waste, especially plastic syringes and needles, were untreated. Overall, large quantities of medical waste were mishandled, with hazardous materials entering the recycling stream and consequently posing a public health risk (Zhao et al., 2009). Following the outbreak, China focused on building waste incineration plants for the purpose of strengthening their medical waste disposal practices and ensuring greater sanitation. While this has led to the improved management of medical waste, a reality demonstrated by China's stronger response to COVID-19, it also means that greater amounts of toxic air pollutants are being emitted to the air. This is ultimately an indirect, long-term response stemming from the SARS outbreak.

4.1.6.3 Changes in the Structure of the Chinese Health Care System

Though China had decided to consolidate its disjointed health care system right before the outbreak of SARS, they chose to model this new organizational structure after the U.S. CDC following the crisis due to its positive global reputation. With a more streamlined, consolidated system, China invested resources into coordinating disease prevention and epidemiological study in order to address emerging infectious disease threats. With renewed public attention on public health and science, the government invested in its newly restructured health care system and began to collaborate more extensively with foreign countries on research, training, and establishing various health programs (Mason, 2020). One of the main long-term changes that took place was the transition from using slower, disorganized outbreak reporting to a more efficient, computerized, real-time surveillance system (Mason, 2020; Huang, 2004). This improved risk communications system likely inherently required the greater use of computers and telecommunications, which have their own impact on global warming and the environment.

Aside from the greater energy usage required by increased computer usage and its associated emissions, a major impact of digitalization in health care is an increase in E-waste due to the fact that computers and mobile telephones have relatively short lifespans. E-waste includes potential environmental contaminants such as lead and cadmium. When E-waste is landfilled, these contaminants can enter into the soil and local water systems, creating a severe public health hazard. These negative environmental impacts are exacerbated by the fact that wealthier countries often export their E-waste to lower-income nations, where fewer regulations and a lack of appropriate recycling technology lead to hazardous disposal through burning and chemical dissolution. Burning generates air pollutants such as polychlorinated biphenyls (PCBs), while the use of strong acids furthers soil and water pollution (Robinson, 2009). Though adequate recycling technology exists, it is expensive. As a result, global recycling of E-waste is not environmentally sustainable, and will continue to get worse, especially as greater telecommunications and computing systems are adopted. Efficient cloud computing networks are becoming more commonplace, which may help offset some E-waste production (Robinson, 2009).

Other long-term changes in China following the SARS outbreak include improved organization of the medical workforce, with greater attention given to improving training on infection control practices and establishing staff designated to emergency risk communication. In addition, coordinated agreements and protocols were establish to overcome administrative hurdles in communications between different arms of the health care sector, including health authorities and medical facilities (Frost et al., 2019). The government also increased funding for improved public health and insurance in rural areas of China, which were seen as weak points in the original failure to contain SARS (Huang, 2004). These effects, however, are beyond the scope of this study.

4.1.6.4 Summary

One of the main changes made to the health care industry in China was a change in methods for proper waste disposal. Prior to the SARS outbreak in China, a large quantity of infectious hospital waste was untreated and mishandled when it came to disposal, leading to hazardous materials entering non-hazardous waste streams, which posed a serious public health risk (Zhao et al., 2009). In response to the outbreak, focus was turned to building new waste incineration plants to improve the sanitation and disposal of hazardous medical waste. While this likely had numerous public health benefits in the long run, another long-term effect that may have stemmed from this was the likely increase of air pollutant emissions in the country. A second major long-term change implemented in response to the SARS outbreak was the digitization of China's risk communication system as a part of the country's decision to modernize and restructure its national health care system. This implies the existence of longer-term impacts related to greater energy usage and E-waste production, which are topics that would benefit from further exploration.

4.1.7 Summary and Populated Framework

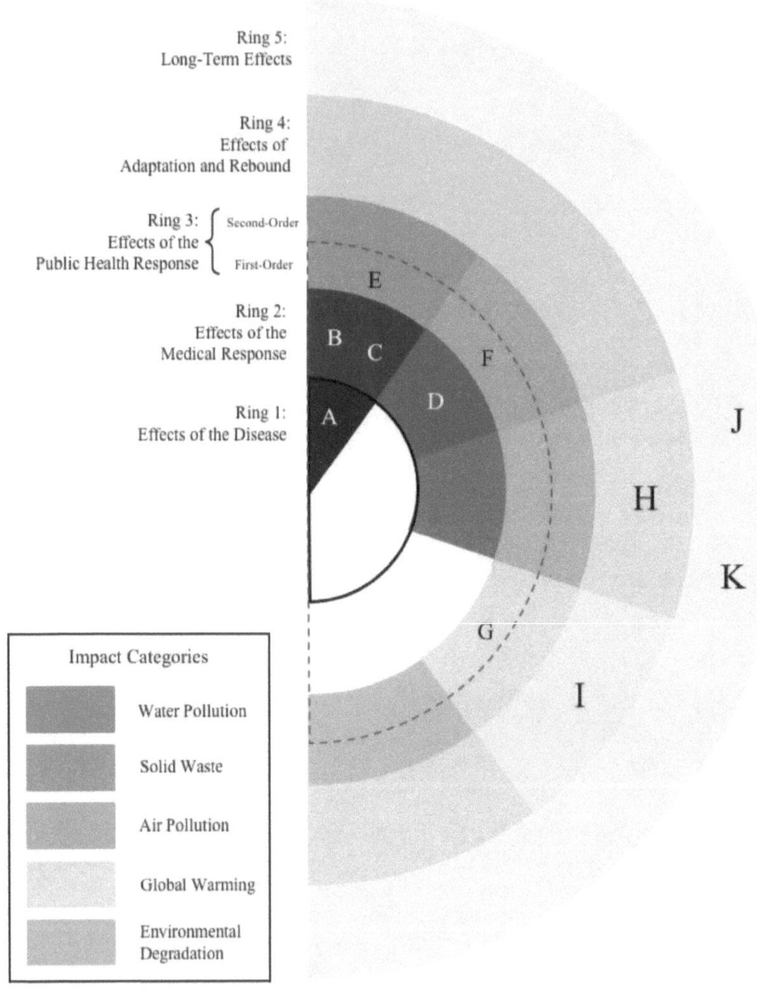

Figure 3. Observed Environmental Impacts of the 2003 SARS Outbreak. Populated through case study application of the developed framework to the SARS outbreak (2003) to assess transferability. Based off of observed environmental impacts and logical conclusions from available literature published in relation to this human health crisis. See Table 2 for corresponding effect descriptions. Note: Figure is not comprehensive.

Table 2: Observed Environmental Impacts of the 2003 SARS Outbreak

	Water Pollution	Solid Waste	Air Pollution	Global Warming	Environmental Degradation
Ring 1: **Effects of the Health Issue**	**A.** Confirmed cases of the presence of the virus in wastewater systems, which could be another source of transmission	No observed effects	No observed effects	No observed effects	No observed effects
Ring 2: **Effects of the Medical Response**	**B.** Probable increase in pollution from antiviral usage **C.** Probable increase in pollution from disinfectant usage	**D.** Increase in medical waste from the treatment of more patients	No observed effects outside of the existing impacts of the health care system	No observed effects outside of the existing impacts of the health care system	No observed effects outside of the existing impacts of the health care system
Ring 3: **First-Order Effects of the Public Health Response**	**E.** Probable increase in water pollution due to disinfectant usage at home and in public spaces	**F.** Increase in plastic waste from greater usage of PPE among citizens	No observed effects	**G.** Plateau in aviation emissions of greenhouse gases such as CO_2 possibly due in part to the outbreak	No observed effects
Second-Order Effects of the Public Health Response	No observed effects	No observed effects	No observed effects	No observed effects	No observed effects
Ring 4: **Effects of Adaptation and Rebound**	No observed effects	No observed effects	**H.** Increase in levels of particulate matter due to investment boom following the outbreak	**I.** Continued increase of aviation emissions after plateau	No observed effects
Ring 5: **Long-Term Effects**	**J.** Changes in the management of solid medical waste: Improved methods for sanitary waste disposal through incineration **K.** Changes in the structure of the Chinese health care system: Improved organizational structure and implementation of digitized risk communications system (Contribution to increased E-waste)				

Addendum:
An additional notable and observed effect that falls under Ring 1 but cannot be adequately classified by existing impact categories:
• Increase in human mortality

Table 2. Summary of Observed Environmental Impacts of the 2003 SARS Outbreak.

63

4.2   Case Study Application #2: New York City Under COVID-19 (2020-2021)

4.2.1   Introduction

In March of 2020, New York City became the center of one of the first major COVID-19 outbreaks in the United States. Though the city reported its first case on March 1st, it is possible that the virus was already circulating in this city and in other U.S. cities (Carey & Glanz, 2020). Between February 29th, 2020 and June 1st, 2020, 203,792 confirmed positive cases and 18,679 deaths were reported to the New York City Department of Health and Mental Hygiene (DOH) (Thompson et al., 2020). During the most intense span of the original outbreak, the city reported a high of 6,578 new (confirmed and probable) cases on April 6th, 2020. The highest 7-day average at this time was 5,449 confirmed and probable cases as of April 7th, 2020. The highest 7-day average for hospitalizations (1,679) was reported on April 4th. The city also reported its highest daily mortality count of 813 confirmed and probable deaths on April 7th (DOH, n.d.-a). On March 22nd, 2020, New York Governor Andrew Cuomo signed the "New York State on PAUSE" Executive Order mandating that all non-essential businesses throughout the state close and temporarily banning all non-essential gatherings of any size, among other directives (New York State, 2020a).

By the end of March, city hospitals were reaching capacity as they struggled to deal with rapidly increasing case counts, and PPE was in short supply (Francescani, 2020). Toward the end of April, cases began to slowly decline, and by June 1st, the 7-day average for new confirmed and probable cases was 629. In New York City, the outbreak eventually became the most subdued by August and September 2020, with the 7-day average for new cases hovering between 250 and 300. By October, however, cases again began to rise in conjunction with the worsening of the pandemic throughout the rest of the country. By January 8th, 2021, the outbreak again reached catastrophic proportions, hitting the highest ever 7-day average for new cases since the beginning of the pandemic at 6,380. New cases peaked on January 4th, 2021 at 7,896, setting another pandemic record for New York City (DOH, n.d.-a). As of April 16th, 2021, New York City has reported over 899,000 total cases since the beginning of its outbreak in March 2020, with roughly 743,000 confirmed cases and 155,000 probable cases (those with a positive antigen test, symptoms and confirmed exposure, or probable death) (DOH, n.d.-b).

New York City was chosen as an additional case study for this paper due to the fact that it can be seen as the original epicenter of COVID-19 in the United States. Strong action by the state government and municipal government occurred over the course of the outbreak, leading to the implementation of focused public health measures. New York City's experience with COVID-19 has provided a chance to explore the use of this study's framework on a smaller scale.

4.2.2 Ring 1: Effects of the Health Issue

4.2.2.1 Introduction

Because this is a localized case study of COVID-19, Ring 1 contains similar findings to those discussed in Chapter 3. This section examines the effects of SARS-CoV-2 on water impacts, human mortality, and reverse zoonotic transmission observed in New York City during 2020. Water impacts discussed in this section are the main environmental finding, but human mortality and reverse zoonosis are also mentioned for their relevance. Findings related to reverse zoonotic transmission were also discussed in Chapter 3 as part of populating the larger framework.

4.2.2.2 Water Impacts

In New York City, the Department of Environmental Protection (DEP) is working with the DOH, as well as other city agencies, to monitor for SARS-CoV-2 in wastewater. The DEP's Bureau of Wastewater Treatment has been continuously collecting samples twice per week from each of its Wastewater Resource Recovery Facilities. Though other studies completed around the world have urged for caution in the possibility of the transmission of the virus via wastewater pathways, the DEP maintains that there is no evidence that SARS-CoV-2 can be transmitted from sewage (DEP, n.d.-a). Throughout the pandemic, increases in traces of the virus were detected in samples from wastewater plants in the boroughs of Brooklyn, Queens, and Staten Island, a trend that coincided with the emergence of COVID-19 hotspots in these areas. As of December, as COVID-19 cases were spiking again, increasing traces of SARS-CoV-2 in wastewater samples started being observed from testing locations throughout the entire city (Kilgannon, 2020). Researchers are hoping that wastewater testing will be a crucial way to track and contain outbreaks due to the fact that increases in the presence of the virus in wastewater can precede an increase in positive test results by anywhere between four to ten days. This is likely due to the fact that infected individuals may excrete high concentrations of the virus before they begin showing symptoms (Tingley, 2020a). For this reason, monitoring sewage concentrations of the virus may be a key factor in alerting public health officials to locations where outbreaks will occur.

4.2.2.3 Human Mortality

As of April 16th, 2021, New York City has reported 32,040 deaths, with roughly 26,968 confirmed and 5,072 probable deaths (cause of death listed as COVID-19 or similar, but with no positive molecular test), putting its mortality rate at approximately 3.6 percent averaged out over the entire pandemic (DOH, n.d.-b). New York City was hit particularly hard during the beginning of the pandemic and suffered a substantial loss of life before communities began to adapt to the disease and learn how to treat it more effectively.

4.2.2.4 Reverse Zoonotic Transmission

As briefly discussed in Chapter 3, instances of reverse zoonotic transmission were reported in New York City at the Bronx Zoo in April of 2020. Overall, eight cats including tigers and lions tested positive for COVID-19 after exhibiting a cough (CDC, 2020a; Wildlife Conservation Society, 2020). While this was the most significant report of reverse zoonotic transmission occurring in the city, it appears that it was an isolated event.

4.2.2.5 Summary

In regard to environmental impacts, there is documented evidence of SARS-CoV-2 within the wastewater system of New York City. The smaller-scale application of this framework allowed for more detailed spatial information regarding wastewater detection of SARS-CoV-2. Traces of the virus have been monitored in numerous boroughs of the city, and some have identified this as an opportunity to detect and contain local community outbreaks before they happen. This is the main way in which the virus itself has impacted New York City's natural environment. Other notable effects of the virus include the substantial loss of life and instances of reverse zoonotic transmission within zoo animals. Though they do not fit into the structure of the framework, they are mentioned for their relevancy to humans and other animals.

4.2.3 Ring 2: Effects of the Medical Response

4.2.3.1 Introduction

As discussed in Chapter 3, the medical response to COVID-19 can largely be characterized through the two main categories of rapid response and treatment. Crucial aspects of this medical response include triage and detection measures, quarantine and isolation protocols within health care facilities, and treatment for those ill with COVID-19. While guidelines were provided by the CDC and other state and municipal health agencies, a significant amount of information on the medical response to New York City's first outbreak of COVID-19 comes from reporting from various hospitals and medical facilities within the city. This is due to the fact that different medical facilities have different organizational structures, supply chains, and are located in different regions with differing populations served, among other discrepancies (Schaye et al., 2020). By looking at the varying responses planned and executed by different health care systems, one can get a more complete picture of how different facilities responded to the outbreak. For example, at four NYU-affiliated hospitals throughout the city, the main challenges faced during the outbreak were ensuring effective communication strategies, developing surge capacity (including allocating proper staffing and implementing adequate triage strategies), determining appropriate clinical care, and maintaining staff wellness (Schaye et al., 2020). In general, the effects of these measures fall under the existing environmental effects of the health care sector discussed briefly in Chapter 3, which are beyond this scope of this study.

4.2.3.2 *Water Pollution*

The review of available news and literature on the COVID-19 pandemic in New York City revealed little to no discussion of water pollution coming directly from pandemic-era medical practices. This may be due to a lack of research focused on this impact area during the pandemic. However, logical conclusions can be made about negative pollution effects of antivirals and disinfectants (even though there is no overt evidence at this time), similarly to how they were made within Chapter 3 and the first case study: In general, disinfectant products can end up in natural water bodies through runoff and through wastewater sewage systems. Common chlorine disinfectants pose a risk to aquatic animals and plants due to the fact that they can damage their cells and bond with other compounds to form highly ecotoxic by-products (Zhang et al., 2020).

4.2.3.3 *Solid Waste*

In New York, regulated medical waste (RMW) is "waste from healthcare facilities contaminated by blood, body fluids, or other infectious materials." The regulation of this waste is managed by the state (New York State Department of Environmental Conservation [DEC], n.d.). In New York State, treatment and disposal of RMW requires a permit, and the state requires this waste to be properly treated and disposed of at an authorized solid waste management facility through autoclaving, incineration, or alternative methods such as microwaving and chemical disinfection. Third-party waste disposal companies are permitted to contract with a waste-producing facility to collect RMW and transport it for disposal at authorized facilities. Waste generators can also be permitted to dispose of RMW in an on-site treatment facility (DEC, n.d.). Thus, in New York State, RMW is overseen at the state level and treated through a decentralized system of medical waste disposal companies. For this reason, there is a lack of encompassing data on changes in medical waste in New York City.

In the U.S., there have been conflicting reports on medical waste generation, which is worsened by the fact that medical waste disposal falls under the jurisdiction of numerous federal agencies, as well as by the fact that legal technicalities result in the differentiation between different types of medical waste and their disposal. In regards to the New York City area, Northwell Health (which serves Westchester County and Long Island in addition to New York City) reported in June 2020 that their 23 hospitals were using 500,000 pairs of gloves per day in comparison to pre-pandemic levels of 250,000 gloves (Doheny, 2020). But while waste output from hospitals stemming from PPE use seemed to increase due to COVID-19, one medical waste disposal company reported that these waste increases could be offset by the decline in elective surgeries (Redling, 2020). Other reports discuss how American waste companies prepared themselves for the high quantities of medical waste seen originally when COVID-19 emerged in Wuhan, China, yet were never met with the expected surge and even saw declines (Brugger, 2020). Therefore, while it can be assumed that the detection and treatment of COVID-19 is increasing medical waste due to the inherent greater need for PPE and other types of equipment, there is a lack of consensus and adequate data on larger medical waste streams overall. There is also a lack of localized data specific to New York City.

4.2.3.4 Air Pollution

As discussed above, regulated medical waste in New York State is treated and disposed of through autoclaving, incineration, or other methods. In New York City, however, the effects of medical waste incineration occurring would likely be negligible due to the fact that conventional waste incinerators are not located within the city limits (New York State, n.d.-a). The last incinerator in the city was torn down in 1999 due to regulations and legislation (Martin, 1999). For the most part, New York City outsources its waste disposal to nearby regions (Goldenberg & Muoio, 2020). As a result, it is crucial to recognize that just because waste incineration does not take place in the city does not mean it is not happening or increasing elsewhere during the pandemic.

4.2.3.5 Summary

Regarding the varied medical response from health care facilities throughout New York City, the framework was applied in order to assess possible effects related to water pollution, solid waste, and air pollution. A review of the literature yielded no overt findings related the medical response in the city and its effect on water pollution. Based on literature discussed in Chapter 3 on the existing impacts of disinfectants and antivirals used in the health care sector, however, it would be reasonable to assume that some of these substances may be ending up in New York City's waterways. At this time, research reviewed specifically for this case study demonstrated no evidence of this due to a lack of focus on this environmental impact area.

Concerning solid waste, New York deals with regulated medical waste through a third-party system in which carting is contracted out to third-party companies. As a result, comprehensive information about large-scale changes in medical waste throughout the city is unavailable. Case-by-case evidence of single health care facilities such as hospitals do demonstrate the likelihood that solid waste production inevitably increased during the pandemic due to the greater usage of PPE. Overall, many factors, such as changes in trends regarding elective surgeries, have complicated this. For this reason, it is difficult to make conclusions about solid waste trends other than the fact that changes have occurred and that RMW in New York City likely increased. Lastly, regarding air pollution, incineration of RMW does not occur within the city due to the fact that there are no facilities located in it that employ this type of disposal method. Direct impacts in this category are therefore virtually non-existent within the city limits. Because New York City outsources its waste disposal, however, incineration practices have simply been moved out of the geography of interest for this case study.

4.2.4 Ring 3: Effects of the Public Health Response

4.2.4.1 Introduction

As discussed at the beginning of this section, on March 22nd, 2020, Governor Cuomo signed an Executive Order mandating the closure of all non-essential businesses throughout the state and temporarily banning all non-essential gatherings of any size. It also established "Matilda's Law" for elderly and other vulnerable populations, directing these groups to remain indoors, refrain from visiting other households, wear a mask around others, and always stay six feet from others, in addition to other measures (New York State, 2020a). This stay-at-home order gave rise to numerous trends in the activity of New Yorkers, many of which had effects on all five categories of water pollution, solid waste, air pollution, global warming, and environmental degradation.

One key trend was the decline in public transportation ridership. At the peak of lockdown in March, the Metropolitan Transportation Authority (MTA) reported that ridership had fallen 87 percent on the subway, 94 percent on the Metro-North commuter rail, 76 percent on the Long Island Rail Road (LIRR), and 60 percent on city buses in one day compared to the same day in 2019 (Yuan & Morgan, 2020). As a result, the MTA had to ask for a $4 billion federal bailout. The decline in public transportation ridership does not necessarily indicate that air pollution and greenhouse gas emissions increased due to the fact that people were staying home, not substituting with driving. Depending on long-term public behavior and sentiment about public health, ridership may remain low, which could lead to long-term effects on air pollution levels or greenhouse gas emissions.

Another policy implemented as part of the public health response to COVID-19 was the DEC's decision to delay the enforcement of New York State's plastic bag ban, which went into effect on March 1st, 2020. Both COVID-19 and an ongoing lawsuit brought by plastic bag manufacturers were the reason enforcement was delayed, but with the end of the lawsuit, it was announced that the ban would begin to be enforced on October 19th, 2020 (WGRZ Staff, 2020). This policy will affect the impact category of solid waste as the continued use of plastic bags over reusable bags has hindered New York City's ability to continue decreasing its solid waste production.

Beyond the delay of the plastic bag ban, it was announced on May 4th, 2020 that the DSNY was temporarily suspending its curbside composting service and other specialty recycling programs until further notice. As a result, residents were asked to discard food scraps and other organic waste into trash (DSNY, 2020). This is another public health policy implemented in response to COVID-19 that directly affected the solid waste category.

The fourth major policy choice implemented was the mandatory use of face coverings and masks in public areas. On April 15th, 2020, Governor Cuomo announced a state order to require residents to wear masks or effective face coverings in public when social distancing is not possible (Ferré-Sadurní & Cramer, 2020). The order applies to those over the age of two who can medically tolerate it. This policy will also influence the waste stream due to the fact that the mandatory usage of face coverings essentially ensures the continued use of disposable face masks, which are discarded into the waste stream after use.

A fifth major policy consideration to be aware of is the current vaccination campaign that began in the winter of 2020 and started expanding in earnest in 2021. As discussed in Chapter 3, vaccines have been authorized for use in combatting against SARS-CoV-2. In the United States, two vaccines were originally approved: the Pfizer-BioNTech vaccine and the Moderna vaccine. (FDA, 2020a; FDA, 2020b). At this time, New York City started to administer these vaccines, starting with health care workers on the front lines. As of April 16th, 2021, the DOH has reported that over 5.5 million doses of any vaccine (including for both the first and second shot) have been administered (DOH, n.d.-c).

4.2.4.2 *Water Pollution*

One key observation noted regarding the category of water pollution under lockdown orders was a short-term improvement in water quality from two factors: greater numbers of individuals staying home and reduced commercial activity. Between March 9th and April 1st, 2020, the analysis of organic and inorganic suspended solids and turbidity taken from satellite data over Manhattan showed a substantial improvement in water quality in the Hudson River, one of the major rivers to flow through New York City. This was due to the fact that fewer people were commuting into the city during the lockdown. Sewage from buildings within New York City is treated in wastewater plants before it is released into the rivers that line the city. With a massive decline in commuters due to the stay-at-home order imposed by New York State, there were fewer people in the city producing these pollutants, and as a result, less was entering the river systems. In one part of the Hudson River, turbidity levels declined by over 40 percent (Bates, 2020). This is a first-order effect due to the fact that it directly resulted from reduced numbers of commuters in the city, which meant that less waste was inherently being produced in this geographic area at the time.

Lastly, it is again notable to mention that as a part of the public health response to COVID-19, sanitation crews have been deployed in New York City throughout the pandemic to disinfect public spaces. For example, in May of 2020, it was announced that the MTA would be halting service in the early morning in order to disinfect every one of its trains (Dwyer, 2020).

This indicates the likelihood that in addition to effects seen as a part of the medical response, disinfectant utilized for this purpose will also likely end up in the city's waterways through runoff and wastewater systems. As discussed, this can have adverse effects on the city's water bodies and the aquatic species that exist in them.

4.2.4.3 Solid Waste: Reporting

Numerous waste trends emerged in New York City following the implementation of stay-at-home orders and some of the other policies discussed above. Within the recycling sector, it was reported by Sims Municipal Recycling (the city's contracted MGP processor) that the volume of metal, glass, and plastic being recycled in April of 2020 increased by 27 percent in comparison to the April average from 2015 to 2019 (Barnard et al., 2020). This is both a first- and second-order effect—more individuals staying home has inherently raised recycling quantities, but with people choosing to order increased take-out from restaurants and purchasing greater quantities of goods through online shopping as a result of staying home, plastic waste is increasing as a second-order effect as well. This comes especially as disposability has been associated with greater sanitation throughout the pandemic, and it is a trend furthered by some of the public health policies discussed above, such as the mask mandate, the delay in the plastic bag ban enforcement, and the implementation of a widespread vaccine campaign. Many of the types of single-use plastics associated with these policies are not recyclable either and must be disposed of through other methods.

On May 4th, 2020, the DSNY announced the temporary suspension of curbside composting service and other specialty recycling programs until further notice. Residents were asked to discard food scraps and other organic waste into their trash (DSNY, 2020). As a first-order result, a significant volume of organic waste is no longer being separated for compost or waste-to-energy pathways. The suspension of compost collection joins hits to other programs such as GrowNYC's zero waste programs and the NYC Compost Project as a part of severe budget cuts made by the Mayor's Office due to the fact that the city hit so intensely by COVID-19. Overall, $28 million dollars were cut from composting programs, education, and outreach as a part of cuts made to the DSNY budget (Peevey & Cohen, 2020).

Regarding residential waste as a whole in the U.S., the general trend seen in many municipalities over the height of their respective lockdown periods was a strong increase in residential waste volumes and declines in commercial waste volumes. This is true for some neighborhoods in New York City, but not for others due to high wealth inequality levels. In April, residential waste declined by 22 percent in the borough of Manhattan, with the highest declines in some of the wealthiest neighborhoods—in Greenwich Village, it declined by 35 percent. This contrasts with waste trends in the city's poorest neighborhoods, where residential waste generally increased—in Morrisania in the South Bronx, it increased by 5.6 percent. Yet, in some of the less dense areas of the city with higher-income single-family households (where there is more outdoor yard space) trash production also increased (Barnard et al., 2020). This disparity is largely due to the fact that wealthier city residents left the city for the suburbs at the beginning of the pandemic. Less wealthy residents, forced to stay home due to lockdown and social distancing measures, accumulated greater quantities of waste at home due to the fact that they were spending more time there. Ultimately, notable changes in waste trends were observed as a first-order effect following the implementation of the heaviest, most restrictive public health policies in New York City resulting from the outbreak of COVID-19. Commercial waste, on the other hand, declined significantly following the implementation of lockdown measures, which was another first-order effect. In less than two weeks following the lockdown, waste from office buildings and business operations fell by 75 percent (Barnard et al., 2020).

4.2.4.4 Solid Waste: Analysis of New York City's Residential Waste Collection (2020)

To conduct an independent analysis of similar trends, monthly residential waste collection data was obtained from the DSNY's public website for the years of 2015 to 2020 (DSNY, n.d.-a). Only residential waste was available due to the fact that the city government is responsible for its collection, while commercial waste is contracted out and hauled by over 90 private carting companies (DSNY, n.d.-b). First, data was consolidated in order to visualize and compare yearly trends for daily tonnage collection by waste category (See Appendix A).

Regarding MGP collection, yearly trends have remained similar, with levels peaking mainly in June and December each year. Over time, MGP collection levels have generally increased (See Appendix A, Figure A-1). Based on the graph, there appears to be a change for the year of 2020, with collection dipping in February and peaking much higher in June. Overall, MGP levels have been much higher in 2020 in comparison to previous years. This is consistent with the increase observed by Sims Municipal Recycling. Paper, on the other hand, has remained fairly steady for the past six years from month to month. There have been some slight variations

73

from year to year, but it doesn't appear that there were any large changes in residential paper collection trends in 2020 during the pandemic (See Appendix A, Figure A-2).

Residential refuse collection has also remained fairly consistent over time, although changes can be observed for the year of 2020. Collection levels for this category dipped down in April before increasing in June and remaining higher than previous years for the rest of the summer (See Appendix A, Figure A-3). Lastly, organics collection has demonstrated a substantial amount of change since it was started in 2013. Since 2015, organics collection levels have steadily increased as more New Yorkers have begun to benefit from the expansion of the program. In 2020, however, when it was announced that curbside organics collection would temporarily stop in May, collection levels fell to nearly zero and remained this way for the rest of the year (See Appendix A, Figure A-4).

To analyze the magnitude of change in residential collection tonnage for the year of 2020, this research adopted the method used by Sims Metal Recycling by calculating the average daily tonnage (for each month) of each category for the years of 2015 to 2019 (See Appendix A, Figures A-5, A-6, A-7, A-8). The calculated quantities for the categories of MGP, paper, and refuse were then compared to the reported 2020 collection quantities for the same months by finding the percentage change between them (See Figure 4) (Note: Organics is not included in Figure 4 because its collection quantities changed significantly over the years of 2015 to 2019). Analysis revealed that the quantity of MGP being recycled during 2020 was higher than 2015-2019 since the beginning of the year. The calculated percentage increase for the month of April was nearly 22 percent, and 29 percent in May. The highest increase occurred in the month of June, when collection was nearly 33 percent higher than it was for the 2015-2019 average. Paper collection in 2020 dipped below the 2015-2019 average in the months of February (-5.69 percent) and April (-8.92 percent), but rebounded to remain above the average from July until October. It reached a high percentage increase of nearly 9 percent in July. Refuse collection demonstrated a similar trend in comparison to its 2015-2019 average, declining by -8.91 percent in April before climbing back up to remain above average from May until December. Refuse collection reached a high percentage increase of 12.6 percent in August.

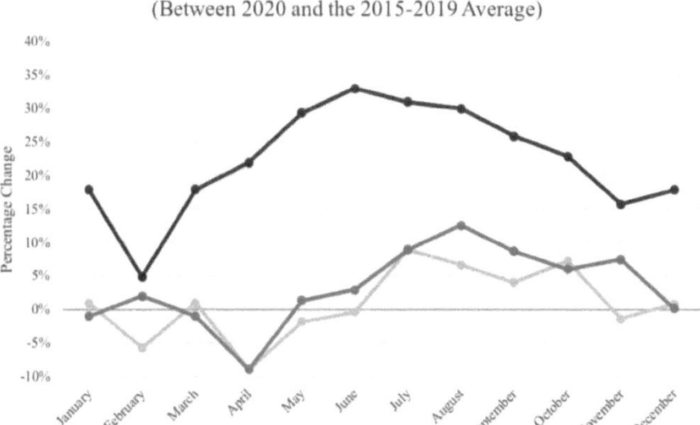

Figure 4. The percentage change in the monthly collection of residential MGP, paper, and refuse in New York City between 2020 and the 2015-2019 average. Data was obtained from the DSNY website.

4.2.4.5 Air Pollution

On March 22nd, 2020, New York was plunged into lockdown after the "New York State on PAUSE" Executive Order from Governor Cuomo mandated the closure of all non-essential businesses and the temporary ban of all non-essential gatherings of any size, among other restrictions. Notable changes in air pollution levels were observed at the height of the lockdown period in New York City as a first-order effect. With more people staying home, it was reported that traffic in the city's busiest areas declined by 60 percent (Hu, 2020). This consequently led to a decline in NO_2 levels and other air pollutants such as $PM_{2.5}$. Zangari et al. (2020) studied daily concentrations of $PM_{2.5}$ and NO_2 from 15 central monitoring stations throughout New York City for the period of January to May for the years of 2015 to 2020. They found that a 36 percent decrease in $PM_{2.5}$ and a 51 percent decrease in NO_2 could be observed in 2020 shortly after the lockdown policies took place. However, the authors used a linear time lag model to compare these results to past years, finding that there was no significant difference. Another study of New York City's pollution emissions estimated a 23 percent decline in $PM_{2.5}$ levels from March 15th to May 15th in comparison to $PM_{2.5}$ levels measured at the same time from 2015-2018 (the

75

business-as-usual period). The researchers did the same for NO$_2$ levels, estimating a 34 percent city-wide reduction in NO$_2$ emissions for the period when compared to 2015-2018 levels (Perera et al., 2021).

4.2.4.6 Global Warming

The decline in traffic levels during the initial lockdown is also applicable to the impact category of global warming. However, at such a localized level, data is not yet available. The City of New York reports on both citywide emissions (from all activities happening within city boundaries) and city government emissions (from all activities associated with government activity) annually through their greenhouse gas emissions inventories (NYC Mayor's Office of Sustainability, 2019). Data for 2020 is not yet available through the city, so it is not possible to definitively claim that greenhouse gas emissions declined following the implementation of lockdown policies. Based on global trends, as well as air pollution and local transportation trends in the city, it can be inferred that emissions likely declined during this time.

4.2.4.7 Environmental Degradation

In recent months, New York City has been dealing with serious issues regarding waste collection due to the fact that the government had to slash the budget of numerous city departments. These department cuts have resulted in fewer collections of public garbage cans and dumpsters. In June of 2020, the city cut the DSNY's budget by $106 million, which caused the collection for public litter baskets to decline by 60 percent. Because of these cuts, residents noted overflowing garbage bins and greater quantities of trash sitting out on the streets for longer periods of time (Bauman, 2020). In addition to the DSNY, the NYC Department of Parks and Recreation's yearly budget was cut by $84 million, or 14 percent. Maintenance crews, which cut the grass, remove weeds, paint over graffiti, and help remove trash, were reduced, leading to 400 fewer parks sites cleaned and 25,000 fewer maintenance hours logged per week (Nir, 2020). These cuts came as many New Yorkers took refuge in parks during the warmer weather, unable to hold social gatherings inside. This, again, resulted in anecdotal evidence of an observable increase in overflowing dumpsters, public waste bins, and garbage strewn all over green spaces (Nir, 2020). This is both a first- and second-order effect due to the combined circumstances of the decreased city budget and more individuals making the conscious choice to go outside to natural areas because of lockdown orders.

4.2.4.8 Summary

As one of the first major locations in the United States to be hit very hard by COVID-19, New York City moved to implement many public health measures in order to prevent the transmission of the virus. Despite the fact that these measures were considered by some to be too little too late as the virus continued to spread to the rest of the country and worsen, these policies did have a serious effect on both daily life and the city's natural environment. The policies implemented and discussed in this section include lockdown orders, a temporary delay in the implementation of the state's plastic bag ban, the suspension of the city's composting collection programs, a mask mandate, and the eventual start of a vaccination campaign as a prevention measure.

The main first-order effect observed in the category of water pollution largely stemmed from the lockdown order implemented by the state government. Emerging data indicates that during the heaviest initial restriction from March to April, water quality improved in the Hudson River, with significant declines in turbidity levels. Because sewage from the city is treated and then released into local waterways, the reduction in activity of people and commuters on shore lead to declines in the production of human waste, which consequently affected the rivers.

Solid waste trends also differed significantly during this time. As both a first and second-order effect, residential MGP recycling quantities increased heavily during lockdown in comparison to recent years. More time spent at home lead to greater overall waste production, while greater delivery of various goods such as take-out orders likely lead to an increase during this time. Organic waste also started being diverted into regular refuse streams due to the fact that the DSNY announced the indefinite suspension of its composting collection service. Through the independent quantitative analysis of New York City's residential collection data conducted for this study, it was found that during 2020, the collection of MGP increased during every month, with collection reaching a high in June of nearly 33 percent higher than it was for the 2015-2019 average. Paper collection in 2020 initially decreased in February and April, but rebounded to remain above the average from July until October. Residential refuse collection additionally declined in April before rebounding to remain above average after May. Organics collection nosedived after the city decided to halt its collection, and it has remained that way since.

On a smaller scale, more nuance was observed in relation to overall residential waste production as well. In numerous wealthy neighborhoods, residential waste declined heavily during the initial lockdown period. At the same time, residential waste increased in many of the city's poorer neighborhoods. This is most easily explained by New York City's burgeoning issues with wealth inequality, where at the time of the lockdown, wealthier residents were able to flee the epicenter of the pandemic and stay elsewhere, while lower-income residents were limited to staying home. But while many people were leaving when the pandemic was at its worst, many of New York's hundreds of thousands of daily commuters were no longer entering the city either. This resulted in commercial waste from office buildings and businesses falling significantly as well.

Air pollution was also seriously affected by the decline in vehicle traffic during the lockdown period. Notable decreases in air pollutants such as NO_2 and $PM_{2.5}$ were observed throughout the city. Because air pollution is linked closely to global warming caused by the emission of greenhouse gases such as CO_2, it can be assumed that this reduction in air pollution also led to a temporary reduction in greenhouse gas emissions. However, because New York City completes its greenhouse gas emissions inventory on a yearly basis, data that proves this is not yet available. While the decline in air pollution from vehicles is a first-order effect, positive global warming effects would fall under both first- and second-order effects due to the fact that energy usage (which contributes to greenhouse gas emissions) is distributed across all aspects of society.

Lastly, much of the city's environmental degradation issues have been related to waste due to the fact that the city itself doesn't have many remote or natural areas other than parks. This is due to city budget cuts as well as the fact that New Yorkers wanted to spend more time outside under strict public health guidelines about indoor gatherings. These cuts led to reduced servicing of public waste bins and dumpsters, and this, combined with increased park usage by individuals, led to anecdotal evidence of trash piling up within the city's parks system. As the only real areas that provide a natural landscape to the city, this is largely the extent of environmental degradation that occurred in New York City during this time.

4.2.5 Ring 4: Effects of Adaptation and Rebound

4.2.5.1 Introduction

Following the initial outbreak and stay at home orders issued by the governor in mid-March, New York State adopted a phased reopening plan as the state continued to deal with and adapt to COVID-19. The governor announced that New York City would be allowed to begin its reopening process for non-essential businesses and business activities on June 8th, 2020 (*Documenting New York's path to recovery…*, n.d.). Industries allowed to resume activities under Phase 1 included construction, agriculture, forestry, fishing and hunting, retail limited to pick-up and drop off services, manufacturing, and wholesale trade (New York State, n.d.-b). The city entered Phase 2 on June 22nd, which allowed for the opening of outdoor dining at bars and restaurants, salons and barbershops, offices, real estate companies, retail, commercial building management, and vehicles sales, leases, and rentals, all with limited capacity to maintain social distancing (*New York Forward Phases,* 2020). The city entered Phase 3 on July 6th, which originally only permitted personal care businesses such as spas and nail salons to reopen and excluded indoor dining (*Documenting New York's path to recovery…*, n.d.; *New York Forward Phases,* 2020). By July 20th, the city entered the final phase (Phase 4) of reopening, which allowed low-risk outdoor arts, entertainment, and recreation to open at 33 percent capacity. Overtime, regulations were slowly expanded to include other aspects of society. It was announced that in-person schooling was expected to reopen in the fall, and other businesses and facilities such as museums, aquariums, and gyms were allowed to open in August. (*Documenting New York's path to recovery…*, n.d.). Indoor dining at 25 percent occupancy was permitted to resume on September 30th (New York State, 2020b).

With the worsening of the pandemic in October, some closures had to occur in order to quell the spread of SARS-CoV-2 in hotspot communities within the city. This was accomplished through a micro-cluster strategy that was applied throughout the entire state and used data to identify and establish temporary zones where infection levels were rising. Depending on the intensity of community outbreaks, these areas have been subject to lockdown restrictions in order to prevent the spread of the outbreak to neighboring communities. Other public health measures as part of this plan included strategies for managing hospital capacity to handle the coming surge of cases, increasing testing, keeping schools open, preventing viral spread through small gatherings, and distributing the vaccine (New York State, n.d.-c).

As the city and state continued to adapt to the COVID-19 pandemic into the winter, the state developed a phased vaccine distribution plan that prioritized the most at-risk community members. Over time, increasing groups of individuals have been added to the eligibility list (New York State, n.d.-d). The city has continued to work with its micro-cluster strategy and vaccine distribution plan in order to slowly try to keep the pandemic under control as it has continued into 2021. The city's adaptation to life during COVID-19 has led to observed and assumed rebounds in certain impact categories as stay-at-home and lockdown orders have been relaxed. These categories include water pollution, solid waste, air pollution, and global warming. A review of the available literature yielded no findings for the category of environmental degradation.

4.2.5.2   Water Pollution

Since original reports of a short-term improvement in water quality in the Hudson River were discussed, little information has since been released on how this may have changed. Analysis of suspended solids and turbidity levels demonstrated that a large decline in commuters in the city led to a decline in wastewater production, which led to improved water quality. Since this time, however, it can be inferred that commuter activity in the city has recovered to a certain extent, with traffic levels in the city having rebounded since March of 2020, a trend that will be discussed more in depth in the air pollution section below (Muoio, 2020). While there are no estimates about how much of this increase in traffic is directly attributable to commuters, it can be assumed that more people are entering the city with the loosening of lockdown restrictions over time. Regarding commuters entering the city via public transportation, ridership levels on some of the major railroads into New York City have shifted slightly. In the first week of March 2021, weekly ridership on the LIRR remained low at roughly 75 percent below 2019 levels, while weekly ridership during the same period on the Metro-North hovered around 80 percent below 2019 levels (MTA, n.d.). This is a slight change in comparison to declines from the peak of lockdown (-76 percent on the LIRR and -94 percent on the Metro-North commuter rail), with the Metro-North having recovered more than the LIRR. Slight recoveries in public transit commuter levels as well as increases in traffic levels indicate that more individuals are entering the city, which has likely cause water quality to begin to decline again. This effect may be furthered by rebounded business activity from companies that utilize the local rivers and waterways of New York City.

As discussed in Ring 3, MGP collection dropped in February with the onset of public health restrictions before recovering during the summer. The percentage increase in MGP collection peaked in June of 2020 at nearly 33 percent and remained significantly higher than the 2015-2019 average for the rest of the year, indicating that as people continued to stay home and adapt under the conditions of the pandemic, demand for recyclable goods or goods packaged in recyclable materials remained high. Paper, which is recycled differently in New York City than MGP, remained fairly similar to the 2015-2019 average throughout the year, dipping by -8.92 percent in April before rebounding to remain above the average from July until October, reaching a high percentage increase of almost 9 percent in July (See Figure 4).

There were stark disparities in how residential waste levels changed immediately after lockdown due to wealth inequality, with waste levels dropping in higher-income neighborhoods due to the fact that people were leaving the city during the worst of the pandemic. The DSNY does not provide localized residential waste collection data that is finer than the borough-level, so the analysis conducted in this paper generalizes by only using the total sum of waste collection throughout the entire city. Overall, the city-wide amount of refuse collected in April of 2020 was -8.91 percent lower than it was during the same period in 2015-2019. By May, however, overall refuse collection had rebounded, and the percentage change in collection between 2020 and the 2015-2019 average remained positive until December. Residential refuse collection reached a high percentage increase of 12.6 percent in August (See Figure 4). In regard to commercial waste levels, continuously depressed commuter levels have kept commercial waste lower than it was in 2019. As of December 2020, industry experts have reported that while commercial waste has made a comeback from the 70 to 90 percent declines seen originally at the beginning of the pandemic, commercial levels have still not rebounded to pre-pandemic levels. This is likely due to the fact that remote work remains prevalent (Khafagy, 2020).

Lastly, the DSNY announced it was suspending organic waste pickup indefinitely in May 2020. During this time, organics collection, which in the beginning of 2020 had been higher than the comparable 2015-2019 average, fell dramatically. Since May, organics collection levels have remained below a daily average of only four tons. At some points throughout the year, organics collection was 98 percent lower than 2015-2019 levels (See Appendix A, Figure A-8).

4.2.5.4 Air Pollution

As discussed in Ring 3, at the beginning of the lockdown period and with the implementation of public health policies aimed at limiting the spread of the virus, both city traffic and ridership levels of public transportation declined. This is significant because vehicles such as cars, buses, and trucks, in addition to being responsible for greenhouse gas emissions, are also responsible for contributing about 11 percent to fine particulate matter and 28 percent to nitrogen oxides levels on a yearly basis in the city (DEP, n.d.). As a result, declines in traffic levels up to 60 percent during the initial lockdown period had pronounced effects on reducing air pollution levels, as discussed in Ring 3. As New York City, along with much of the world, began adapting to life under the pandemic, it was reported in September of 2020 that driving was rebounding faster than public transportation ridership. In comparison to pre-pandemic levels, traffic in the city's busiest areas (bridges and tunnels) was only down an average of 18 percent (compared to 60 percent in April). At the same time, however, subway ridership was still reported to be down an average of 78 percent in comparison to 2019, while bus ridership was still down by 50 percent (Muoio, 2020).

This is supported by Apple, Inc.'s mobility data, which shows that driving and transit trends nosedived in New York City in March and April. By the late summer, however, driving had rebounded to levels that were higher than pre-pandemic levels, likely due to the fact that as people adjusted to the pandemic and stay-at-home orders were lifted, people began to travel more, but preferred using their cars to avoid public contact. Driving trended downward, however, and is now again below pre-pandemic baseline levels as of January and February 2021. Transit, on the other hand, has yet to recover from its rapid decline at the beginning of the pandemic—since March, it has remained low at about 50 percent below pre-pandemic levels (*COVID-19 Mobility Trends Reports,* n.d.). Even with persistent depressed trends in transit, the fact that driving levels have rebounded is an indication of a rise in air pollution levels. This is documented—by December of 2020, air quality reports from the DOH have shown that NO_2 levels from one monitoring area have rebounded back to pre-pandemic 2019 levels (*New York's Next Comeback,* 2020).

4.2.5.5 Global Warming

The transportation trends discussed in the above section are equally applicable to the impact category of global warming. Public transportation in New York City has long been responsible for limiting greenhouse gas emissions levels—it helps the city avoid roughly 17 million metric tons of emissions per year (Muoio, 2020). Traffic from vehicles, however, is a significant contributor to the city's greenhouse gas emissions. As the pandemic has worn on, this reality has become a problem as city car travel has resurged (and is now down by only 18 percent in comparison to pre-pandemic levels) while public transportation ridership has remained more depressed (subway ridership is down by 78 percent while bus ridership is down 50 percent in comparison to 2019 levels). Though city data is not yet available on greenhouse gas emissions, the increase in vehicle traffic has led to both a rebound in local air pollution and a likely rebound in greenhouse gas emissions.

4.2.5.6 Summary

Like much of the world, New York City has gone through hills and valleys of the COVID-19 pandemic, with major waves of infections occurring in March and April and from October through the winter months into 2021. Throughout this time, state and city leaders have had to adjust their public health policies to respond to outbreaks and keep cases as low as possible. Over time, however, the city saw a gradual loosening of policies, even when cases began rising again and causing localized closures and restrictions. With this gradual reopening throughout the adaptation part of this stage, numerous changes have occurred that are documented within the framework's environmental impact categories.

In regard to water pollution, there is no direct evidence that the gains in water quality made under lockdown have vanished yet. At the same time, vehicle traffic was reported to increase again through a slow rebound, along with a slight improvement in ridership of the city's commuter trainlines. As a result, it is reasonable to assume that certain levels of human activity within the city have increased with the return of some commuters. In consequence, water pollution levels have likely begun to increase again with greater human waste being produced, treated, and discharged into local waterways within the city.

In relation to solid waste, little information was available within the literature on how these trends changed over time as the city adjusted to life under the pandemic and started to implement its phased reopening program. This was where the quantitative analysis conducted for this study became especially useful. As discussed above, it was found that during 2020, collection of MGP had increased during every month in comparison to the 2015-2019 average. This category reached a maximum increase in June before slowly declining, but throughout

2020, it remained above the previous average collection levels. As city inhabitants adjusted, paper collection, which had originally decreased in February and April, eventually rebounded and remained above the 2015-2019 average from July until October. Similarly, refuse collection had declined in April, but rebounded as well and remained above average from May until December. Since the city postponed its composting collection service in May of 2020, organics collection declined severely and has remained negligible since.

4.2.6   Ring 5: Long-Term Effects

4.2.6.1   Introduction

COVID-19's effect on New York City during 2020 was severe, leading to such a significant disruption in life and business that it was common to hear calls of how parts of the city, such as Midtown Manhattan, would never be the same again. The long-term effects of COVID-19 in this region have yet to be seen in full, but a few notable trends and suggestions have emerged as the city continues to work on managing its caseloads and preventing outbreaks. As a dense center of economic life, some are rethinking how this space can best be repurposed to support both the environment and responsible public health practices, while others are examining how COVID-19 may change long-term commuting trends. There are questions about migration trends seen during the thick of the pandemic, and there are indications that long-term stress on the city government's financial system may harm the maintenance of valuable programs such as composting. As these effects continue to play out, it is difficult at this time to make conclusions, but presented below are some of the possible long-term effects that may result in the aftermath of the COVID-19 pandemic. These effects could have serious implications for the natural environment.

4.2.6.2   Changes in Long-Term Waste Trends

Though organic composting collection was originally suspended indefinitely, by November 2020, the city announced that curbside compost collection would be halted until at least June 30th, 2022. As a result, large amounts of waste that could have been diverted to more sustainable pathways such as waste-to-energy production or become natural fertilizer for city parks will end up within the city's waste stream for a prolonged period of time. In addition, cuts to composting programs within the city have eliminated green jobs in organics recycling, may hinder the city's ability to meet its climate goals, and will worsen greenhouse gas emissions in the long-run due to the fact that more organic matter will be sent to rot and produce methane in landfills (Peevey & Cohen, 2020)

4.2.6.3 Changes in Environmental Maintenance

Due to the fact that numerous city departments such as the DSNY and the Parks Department have suffered severe budget cuts under the pandemic's financial strain on the city, it will take time for them to recover and regain momentum when it comes to many environmentally-beneficial programs. The fiscal crisis facing the city at the moment has serious implications for the city moving forward (*New York's Next Comeback,* 2020). As a result, parks and public spaces in the city may remain observably dirtier than they were before the pandemic. A lack of money and the manpower necessary to keep the city clean may persist as the government focuses on what it deems to be more important short-term initiatives.

4.2.6.4 Changes in Transportation

It is also estimated that long-term behavior change surrounding New York City's public transportation system may remain long after the pandemic is declared over. The Regional Planning Association, a non-profit urban planning organization that focuses on the New York metropolitan area, has estimated that if Manhattan gains just two-thirds of the jobs it has lost, there's a chance that 25 percent more people will choose to drive to work in comparison to pre-pandemic levels while public transportation ridership will remain depressed (Muoio, 2020). In addition, due to the fiscal crisis, public services suffered throughout 2020, threatening the long-term maintenance of the city's infrastructure and public transportation system (*New York's Next Comeback,* 2020). Should the decline of the city's public transit system occur, this will disproportionately harm low-income communities as well as the environment due to the fact that these services are crucial to reducing the city's air pollution and carbon emissions.

At the same time, however, this past year has seen the introduction of numerous state and city policies designed to reduce vehicle traffic and encourage zero carbon transportation modes such as biking. In September 2020, New York City Mayor Bill de Blasio announced that the Open Streets program, which began last spring, would eventually become permanent. This program closed certain streets to traffic to provide pedestrians with more room to adhere to social distancing norms while enjoying outdoor activities (*NYC Open Streets...,* 2020). In February, he expanded on this, adding that the city would work to expand protected bike lanes by creating "Bike Boulevards" in every borough and creating additional pedestrian and bike lanes on the Queensboro and Brooklyn Bridges. The city's Department of Transportation has additionally stated that it will install 10,000 bike parking racks in the city by the end of 2022 (Griffin, 2021). On March 5th, 2021, Governor Cuomo additionally announced that $5 million would be awarded to the Hudson River Park Trust in order to construct a new pedestrian and bike path in Manhattan (New York State, 2021). Should these measures successfully take effect, this could have an impact on lowering both greenhouse gas emissions and local air pollution.

4.2.6.5 *Changes in Urban Space*

As previously discussed, in September 2020, Mayor Bill de Blasio announced the permanent establishment of the Open Streets program, which will close some streets to traffic (*NYC Open Streets...*, 2020). Beyond its relation to transportation, this shows potential for long-term change in how the city decides to approach urban space. A shift towards urban planning that accommodates social distancing and health precautions will also lead to greater health and climate benefits that come from reduced vehicle congestion in a repurposed space. This connects to ideas emerging in architecture about not only building and transforming urban spaces to be more inclusive and environmentally friendly, but also more beneficial for public health (Tingley, 2020b).

Another example of long-term change that may take place relates to the commercial sector. 2020 saw the steep decline of New York City's commercial real estate industry, with 14 percent of office space in Midtown Manhattan becoming unoccupied. As a result, some landlords are pushing the city to allow them to more easily convert their properties into housing facilities (Haag & Rubenstein, 2020). Should this happen, this will likely change the fabric of the city due to Midtown's long history as a center of business. At this point, the environmental effects that may result from a change like this are unknown.

4.2.6.6 *Changes in City Life and Movement to the Suburbs*

In Chapter 3, it was discussed that the fear of human density in daily life may be pushing wealthier families to move towards the suburbs (Florida et al., 2020). In July 2020, there were reports of New York City residents moving to the suburbs, and suburban real estate agents were noting higher numbers of inquiries and offers for properties surrounding the city (Berliner, 2020). One moving company interviewed by the New York Times reported that the number of moves it completed between March and August of 2020 had increased by over 46 percent compared to the same period the year before. The company reported a 50 percent increase in those moving outside of New York City, which accounted for a 232 percent increase to Dutchess County and a 116 percent increase to Ulster County, two counties located north of the city in the Hudson Valley (Satow, 2020). In July, home sales were up by 44 percent in the counties around the city while Manhattan sales were down by 56 percent (*New York's Next Comeback,* 2020). Though there is indication that the decline in city residents is partially temporary, with some already coming back, low tax revenues and fiscal strain due to the pandemic, continued high housing prices, and an aging transportation system could point to this exodus remaining a long-term trend (*New York's Next Comeback,* 2020).

4.2.6.7 *Summary*

Many of New York City's long-term environmental effects from COVID-19 are yet to be seen in full due to the fact that the pandemic is still ongoing. Despite this, multiple policy decisions have already set some in motion. This section discusses the long-term implications of the city's budget cuts, which include slashes to the funding for its organic waste program and parks maintenance. The long-term postponement and decline in funding for the city's curbside composting pickup service will not only influence solid waste streams in the future, but could have broader effects on the city's ability to meet climate goals. In addition, cuts to the city's Parks Department will hinder the department's ability to staff enough crews to maintain green spaces within the city.

Many other possible long-term effects concern the movement and migration of people. Notably, changes in transportation trends may occur in the long-term. As the pandemic has wound on, public transit ridership has remained depressed, rebounding at a far slower pace in comparison to vehicle traffic. This may indicate that in the future, people in New York City may increasingly prefer to drive rather than take public transportation. Because public transportation plays a crucial role in lowering the city's greenhouse gas emissions, this may harm the city's progress in regard to lowering its transportation sector emissions in the long-run. These trends may be counteracted by increased efforts by the city and state government to open more city streets up to pedestrian traffic and support initiatives to encourage greater cycling within the city as an alternative to other means of transportation.

Other possibilities for long-term change include modifying the way city residents and companies use public space. Greater emphasis is being put on opening congested areas and using architecture to accommodate growing public health concerns. On a more concrete level, other spaces may be shifting in purpose, with property owners in Midtown Manhattan pushing zoning officials to allow them to convert commercial spaces into residential apartments. This is occurring as COVID-19 gave way to increased trends in residents moving out of the city. While there is evidence that this may be a temporary trend, numerous factors may exacerbate this and lead to a longer-term exodus of New Yorkers. Overall, many of these possibilities are speculative and cannot yet be tangibly documented. However, should some of these occur, they will likely have significant effects on environmental factors such as energy consumption, waste streams, pollution, and many more. Further research will be needed in the years to come in order to fully understand some of the reverberating changes that may be happening in New York City.

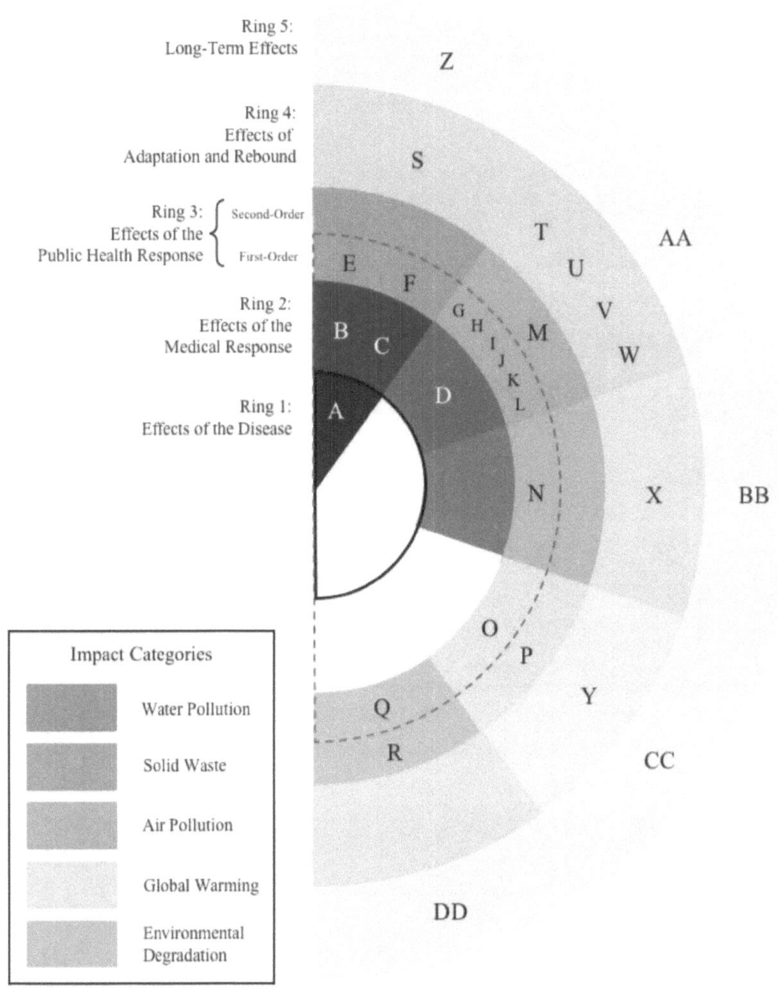

Figure 5. Observed and Expected Environmental Impacts of the COVID-19 Pandemic in New York City. Populated through case study application of the developed framework to New York City to assess scalability. Based off of observed environmental impacts and logical conclusions from available literature published in relation to New York City's experience with this human health crisis. See Table 3 for corresponding effect descriptions. Note: Figure is not comprehensive.

Table 3: Observed and Expected Environmental Impacts of the COVID-19 Pandemic in New York City					
	Water Pollution	**Solid Waste**	**Air Pollution**	**Global Warming**	**Environmental Degradation**
Ring 1: **Effects of the Health Issue**	A. Confirmed cases of the presence of the virus in wastewater systems, which could be another source of transmission	No observed effects	No observed effects	No observed effects	No observed effects
Ring 2: **Effects of the Medical Response**	B. Probable increase in pollution from antiviral usage C. Probable increase in pollution from disinfectant usage	D. Probable increase in medical waste from the treatment of more patients, though it may be partially offset by a reduction in elective procedures	No observed effects outside of the existing impacts of the health care system	No observed effects outside of the existing impacts of the health care system	No observed effects outside of the existing impacts of the health care system
Ring 3: **First-Order Effects of the Public Health Response**	E. Decline in water pollution from reduction in commuter activity F. Probable increase in water pollution due to disinfectant usage in public spaces	G. Increase in metal, glass, and plastic (MGP) waste H. Diversion of residential organic waste to residential refuse flows I. Variable shifts in residential waste production as part of overall decline in April 2020 J. Decline in commercial waste production due to lockdown K. Decline in residential paper waste production in April 2020 L. Probable increase in medical waste due to eventual improper vaccine disposal	N. Short-term decline in NO_2 and $PM_{2.5}$ pollution from reduction in mobility	O. Probable short-term decline in emissions of greenhouse gases such as CO_2	Q. Increase in pollution of natural spaces due to maintenance budget cuts resulting from the COVID-19 economic crisis
Second-Order Effects of the Public Health Response	No observed effects	M. Increase in plastic waste from disposable packaging	No observed effects	P. Probable short-term decline in emissions of greenhouse gases such as CO_2	R. Probable increase in pollution of natural spaces due to greater public park patronage during lockdown period
Ring 4: **Effects of Adaptation and Rebound**	S. Expected reversal in water pollution reductions from rebounded activity	T. Continued increase of MGP waste collected over the summer U. General rebound and increase in paper waste collected over the summer V. General rebound and increase in refuse collected for the rest of 2020 W. General rebound in commercial waste, though not to pre-pandemic levels	X. Reversal in air pollution reductions	Y. Expected reversal in short-term greenhouse gas emissions declines	No observed effects
Ring 5: **Long-Term Effects**	Z. Changes in long-term waste trends: Long-term decline in organic waste collection possible due to government policies. AA. Changes in environmental maintenance: Cuts to city department budgets may hinder the ability to keep public spaces clean. BB. Changes in transportation: Commuter shift from public transportation to driving; Policies and increased economic support for city biking and pedestrian traffic CC. Changes in urban space: Future use of urban planning practices and architectural design to incorporate inclusivity, environmental considerations, and public health; Transformation of business districts in the heart of the city into neighborhoods with housing DD. Changes in city life and movement to the suburbs: Possible long-term migration out of city due to desire for more space and perceived better public health conditions				

Addendum:
Additional notable and observed effects that fall under Ring 1 but cannot be adequately classified by existing impact categories:
- Increase in human mortality
- Cases of reverse zoonotic transmission

Table 3. Summary of Observed and Expected Environmental Impacts of the COVID-19 Pandemic in New York City (2020-2021).

Chapter 5: Discussion, Implications, and Conclusions

5.1   Introduction

The purpose of developing this framework and applying it to different scenarios was to assess how the COVID-19 pandemic has revealed the far-reaching effects that a human health crisis can have on the environment. As a natural experiment of unprecedented scale, it provided the opportunity to explore how a large-scale pause in human activity in conjunction with an active global public health campaign can influence numerous categories of environmental impacts and how this improved understanding may be applied in the future to better bridge the environment-public health knowledge gap. Chapter 3 consisted of cataloguing the observed and expected environmental effects of the pandemic (bolstered by existing impacts of human health on the environment) in order to develop a framework. In Chapter 4, this framework was applied through two case studies to assess its strengths and weaknesses. The first case study focused on a past human health crisis, the 2003 SARS outbreak, which provided an opportunity to explore the framework's adaptability for use in other scenarios. This case study provided numerous insights, including the idea that the framework is effective in pointing out areas of environmental impacts that may be hidden, especially when applied to a case that has a weaker public health response. A second case study was then conducted by applying the framework to assess the COVID-19 crisis on a smaller scale. New York City was chosen for this case study for its status as the original epicenter of the pandemic in the United States. This study provided insights that differed from the findings of the SARS case study, including the fact that scaling down analysis leads to the cutoff of larger-scale impact pathways while also providing an opportunity to analyze more granular trends in data. The main findings from Chapters 3 and 4 are presented below.

5.2   Discussion of Chapter 3 Findings

Finding #1: For Ring 1, there are some opportunities for improvement due to the fact that it includes effects that do not fit into the established categories of the framework. This framework was structured by basing it off of the idea of what we as humans stereotypically think of as impacts on the natural world—water, waste, air, and natural ecosystems. But as shown in this section, there are other impacts that can toe the line of impacting the "natural world." In this case, human mortality and reverse zoonotic transmission of the disease were either too severe or too relevant to ignore while conducting the literature review for this study. This ring ultimately shows how it can be difficult to navigate separating humans and human activity from nature itself—when thinking about what people typically consider pristine nature, it is uncommon to think of humans. In the end, however, humans are another species on Earth. The same goes for reverse zoonotic transmission. Most cases of reverse zoonosis occurred in animals that were in captivity. Though some cases occurred in what we consider wild animals, such as tigers, it begs the question: If they're in captivity, do they at any point cease to be a part of what we consider "the natural world?" This research does not attempt to answer this question. Rather, this is something to consider when trying to improve upon this framework.

Finding #2: Ring 2 indicates that there is room for greater research into water contamination from the medical field. In Ring 2, which dealt with the medical response, assumptions were made about disinfectant and antiviral pollutants in regard to COVID-19. These were based off of existing peer-reviewed literature that proves the negative aquatic effects of these substances on natural water bodies. At the time of research, a review of the literature yielded no specific studies related to disinfectant or antiviral loading of aquatic compartments during COVID-19. This may be due to the fact that research could still be emerging on this topic due to its novelty, but it could also be a sign that analysis of water contamination may be a weak research topic in the area of public health and environmental pollution. This may present a greater opportunity for a research focus in the future.

Finding #3: Ring 4 provides a general structure with which to assess the effects of adaptation and rebound but more time is needed to make conclusions. The population of Ring 4, adaptation and rebound, in Chapter 3 was weak due to time constraints related to the study—because COVID-19 was happening concurrently, it was difficult to populate this impact stage of the framework while adaptation was underway. As a result, this ring's contributions in Chapter 3 are limited. The most important role the establishment of this ring played was providing a lens through which to examine the case studies, which are presented in Chapter 4. These case studies build on the structure established by this ring and demonstrate that adequate time is needed to improve on the assessment of the adaptation and rebound stage of a human health crisis. Case studies using this framework will be best-conducted when enough time has elapsed in order to more fully assess how a region or society as a whole may bounce back from a human health crisis. This was ultimately proven through the SARS case study—with more time to look at the trends documented in the literature following the SARS outbreak in Asia, more complete conclusions could be made about the findings for Ring 4 in this study.

Finding #4: Ring 5 demonstrates how reverberating effects from an event of such a massive magnitude can abstract into ideas that very clearly move beyond framework classification. While most effects discussed in this impact stage have not been thoroughly explored within the literature, many early ideas have emerged about the ways in which COVID-19 and its subsequent medical and public health responses may affect the world in the long-run. For this reason, Ring 5 is more loosely structured than the other rings, which provides more leniency when using the framework to account for long-term possibilities. These ideas are important to include because they may have profound implications for how we think about the interaction between human health crises and the environment. For this reason, further research is required in the future to adequately understand these effects.

Finding #5: The environmental impact category of environmental degradation is broad and could perhaps benefit from being refined. This category has the potential to be separated into two or more categories, with possibilities for classifications related to biodiversity, ecotoxicity, natural resource consumption, and eutrophication, among others. The idea of establishing environmental degradation as an impact category was to account within the framework for harm happening to natural ecosystems. Because ecosystems can be affected through a multitude of different ways, more specificity regarding this impact category could be pursued in the future.

5.3 The SARS Outbreak: Discussion of Findings

Finding #1: A lack of technology and communications as well as a lack of societal focus on environmental issues at the time of the outbreak led to weaker environmental coverage of SARS in comparison to the COVID-19 pandemic. During the outbreak, much of the focus fell on maintaining public health, while with COVID-19, more nuanced observations have been made regarding some of the pandemic's environmental impacts (in addition to the non-stop coverage of public health). As a result, in completing this case study, finding more specific data related to the impact categories was difficult. This ultimately led to the inability to draw conclusions about some impact areas of the framework.

This was particularly apparent in Rings 3 and 4. With the public health response, very little information was found in relation to effects on air pollution or environmental degradation, and possible effects related to water pollution and solid waste were based off of assumptions from public health guidelines—for example, certain areas recommended the use of bleach to disinfect one's home or required masks to prevent the spread of the virus. For this reason, one could assume that local waterways and waste streams were likely affected. However, there is no overt evidence in the literature of this occurring, and there is no way to assess the magnitude of these affects. This shows that while the framework is helpful for pointing out possibilities for environmental effects, it is currently not equipped to help prove them or quantify them. It also does not necessarily guarantee that effects will be there.

This was also the case for Ring 4 of this case study. In general, observed effects about the adaptation to and rebound from the SARS outbreaks were highly limited. Some information about rebounding air pollution and greenhouse gas emissions was found within the literature, but overall, water pollution, solid waste, and environmental degradation were not studied within the literature during this impact stage of the outbreak. This demonstrates that the framework may run into difficulty when applied to other health crises, especially when the adaptation and rebound stage occurs much more rapidly.

Finding #2: The framework provides a useful roadmap for examining possible effects. While the sparse data available shows an aspect of the framework's weakness, the lack of information simultaneously demonstrated how the framework can excel in revealing impacts that may otherwise stay hidden. In conducting the case study on a crisis whose academic coverage included little discussion of its environmental impacts, the framework actually provided valuable direction on where to look for impacts that might have occurred at the time. In conducting this case study, a search of scholarly sources and news was carried out for each impact stage and environmental impact category within the framework. During this time, looking for possible air pollution impacts resulting from the medical response to SARS yielded no direct findings. It did, however, reveal that though waste incineration methods for the disposal of hazardous medical waste were not common in China before the SARS outbreak, the health crisis catalyzed a response that led to the increase of attention toward improving the country's proper disposal of medical waste, indicating a possible long-term environmental effect that was observed in Chapter 3 (China now uses waste incineration plants to dispose of some of its hazardous medical waste). Thus, though some environmental impacts may not have been recorded in connection with the outbreak, the understanding of a human health crisis provided by the framework pointed out connections that were not recognized at the time.

Finding #3: The SARS outbreak demonstrates how a less drastic public health crisis will not fully populate the framework when it is applied. Some environmental impact categories were not influenced during the SARS outbreak due to the fact that less restrictive public health policies were implemented for a shorter period of time. From this, it can be concluded that the most significant environmental impacts stemming from a human health crisis are a result of the severity and expansiveness of the public health policies enforced during them. Because lockdown measures and travel restrictions were not as intense during this outbreak, human movement and activity were not as limited as they have been during COVID-19. For this reason, environmental impacts during the SARS outbreak were seemingly not as intense. This also indicates that for this framework to function to its fullest extent, it may require more intense conditions, which is why its applicability to analyzing other human health crises may be hindered. If applied to a future health crisis, it may be difficult to fully populate and will act as a structure for the possibilities of the impacts that could occur in a given scenario.

5.4 COVID-19 in New York City: Discussion of Findings

Finding #1: Scaling down the application of the framework can lead to the cutoff of larger-scale regional flows of impact. In New York City, trends such as a decline in residential waste were observed in certain neighborhoods as a result of public health measures requiring individuals to stay home at the beginning of the pandemic. Upon further research, it became clear that this was occurring due to the fact that wealthier New Yorkers were leaving the city for the suburbs during the worst part of the pandemic. As a result, the waste generated by this group of people was taken to a geographic region outside of New York City. The same logic applies to air pollution in Ring 2 of this case study. Air pollution effects related to medical waste incineration were not observed as part of this impact stage, but this was due to the fact that incineration does not occur within New York City. Medical waste is exported, where it is incinerated or treated elsewhere. Therefore, both of these examples show how this framework can be misleading without an understanding of the broader context—waste generation didn't necessarily decline, it just moved elsewhere. Thus, while a smaller-scale application can reveal how environmental impacts are occurring locally, it will not account for how changes may be occurring in a broader region. This consequently demonstrates a weakness of this framework in terms of its scalability—on a more granular level, the framework does not account for the impact flows that may be entering and exiting this region's environment. This drawback in scalability of the framework, which will likely occur at any scale other than the global level, is a factor that can be improved upon through the future development of this framework.

Finding #2: Using a scaled down, more-focused application of the framework allows for sharper analysis of community trends in environmental impacts. By focusing on a small geographic region instead of the entire world, small-scale application of the framework can provide a robust structure for analyzing how local trends in environmental impacts respond through each stage of a human health crisis. For example, spatial analysis of New York City's waste trends at the height of its lockdown revealed that certain higher-income neighborhoods saw declines in residential waste while other lower-income neighborhoods saw increases. The quantitative research conducted in Ring 3 of this case study, on the other hand, found that overall residential waste collection declined below average in April before increasing to above average levels over the summer. Analyzing a smaller geographic area allows for more granular discrepancies to be observed in trends that would otherwise be generalized or muddled by increasing influencing factors on a larger level.

Finding #3: While an organized government entity can provide useful information, case-specific decentralization of data collection can lead to major gaps in analysis. Overall, the purpose of the framework and its application through case studies is not to account for every single effect that may be occurring. But because the application of the framework does necessitate looking for and cataloging some effects, the process does expose gaps whereby a lack of consolidated data can complicate the understanding of an impact category. This conclusion is a result of research and analysis performed on solid waste trends in Ring 3. The City of New York provided useful data for analysis on residential solid waste collection, which helped reveal insights about longer-term trends that have occurred throughout the city's adaptation to the pandemic. Analysis of commercial waste, on the other hand, was not possible due to the fact that this waste sector is contracted out, with commercial collection all over the city carted by over 90 private waste companies (DSNY, n.d.-b). As a result, the decentralization of commercial waste collection made it impossible to obtain comprehensive data for analysis of waste produced by this sector at the time this study was conducted. While this may not be the case in other municipalities or cities elsewhere, the lack of consolidated data and information available on an impact category may lead to difficulty drawing conclusions on such a granular level of analysis when using this framework.

5.5   Implications

Overall, this research has the potential to improve how we assess human health crises moving forward. As shown by the first case study of the 2003 SARS outbreak, it is clear that the theoretical framework developed by this research can be used in future applications to broadly assess the impacts of human health and a health crisis response on the environment. The second case study on COVID-19 in New York City also demonstrates that this framework can be adapted for use on non-global scales. While this framework can be improved in the future, it still successfully offers an introductory method for taking a more expansive approach in understanding the environmental connections to a human health crisis. By taking a wider lens, this may enable us to better understand how public health is inherently tied to our natural environment, and it may aid us in better preparing for a health crisis in the future by closing the environment-public health knowledge gap.

5.6   Limitations of Current Research

This research was largely limited by the fact that COVID-19, which was used to populate most of the framework, was occurring concurrently. Because of this, information and data available kept changing throughout the research process. As a result, the inductive formation of the theoretical framework presented in this paper had to be adaptable and fluid. In addition, this paper was completed within a limited time frame, resulting in limited exploration into certain effects that could have larger implications for the framework. With more time and resources, this framework could be expanded. Lastly, discussion of the findings of this research revealed that there is room for improvement within the structure of the framework itself—categories can be refined, theoretical pathways can be introduced to help account for exiting and entering impact flows, and overall improvements can be made to enable the framework to more comprehensively account for quantifiable results.

5.7   Suggestions for Future Research

The most crucial way in which this research can be applied is to continue using it to catalog and analyze long-term effects of the COVID-19 pandemic. Long-term effects within this research were largely speculative due to the fact that the pandemic is ongoing. With time, this framework could be used to help account for some of the trends related to the environmental impacts of COVID-19 in the long run. The further population of this framework from COVID-19 will only serve to improve and strengthen it. Additional research could focus on using just one section or aspect of the framework to take a deeper look at trends related to one impact category or stage, such as waste trends resulting from the public health response. This process could be used to identify possible sub-categories that could be utilized. Overall, the framework should continue to be applied and tested through further case study application in order to continue identifying its strengths and weaknesses.

5.8   Conclusion

The original aim of developing this framework was to aid researchers in taking a more interdisciplinary, systems-based approach to assessing how a human health crisis can affect the natural environment. It was created, based off of, and populated from COVID-19, one of the most significant human health crises in recent history. Overall, numerous environmental impacts have been observed throughout the five impact stages of the pandemic. Regarding the disease itself, the virus was found within wastewater systems, indicating its circulation through natural water bodies. The medical response was characterized by an increase in solid medical waste from the treatment of patients and a probable increase in water pollution from the usage of antivirals in treatment and disinfectant in health care facilities.

Some of the most significant environmental impacts of the pandemic have stemmed from the widespread public health response that has taken place, which included the enforcement of lockdown orders and travel restrictions across the globe. Reductions in human activity during this time led to impacts such as declines in water pollution from reduced recreational and industrial activity, short-term declines in air pollution and greenhouse gas emissions from reduced transportation, and declines in environmental disturbance due to stay-at-home orders. Increases in plastic waste were observed as a result of the widespread wearing of face masks and the greater utilization of disposable packaging to ensure sanitation during this time. As effects of human mobility restrictions rippled across every aspect of society, numerous other impacts emerged, including an increase in organic waste from halted agricultural exports, a short-term increase in ground-level ozone pollution, and a decline in environmental protection due to the reduction of environmental monitoring and ecotourism.

As society began to adapt to the reality of life under a long-term pandemic, however, many of the beneficial environmental impacts observed from a reduction in human activity soon began to reverse. Water pollution was expected to begin increasing again, air quality improvements have declined due to a rebound in transportation, and greenhouse gas emissions reductions observed at the height of the lockdown have additionally rebounded with the eventual increase in human activity. Though environmental monitoring has returned in many regions, increased park patronage has led to pollution of natural areas, and the pervasive use of face masks throughout society is an indication that medical waste will continue to show up in the natural environment, polluting ecosystems and harming the species within them.

Lastly, many long-term changes may pervade throughout society long after the pandemic is considered over. Behavioral changes may lead to a long-term decline in the trust of public transportation, a preference for digital services and remote work, and the increase in movement out of cities and into suburban areas. Long-term changes may occur in regard to international cooperation and climate policy, urban geography, transportation, and economic activity and business. All of these changes will impact various aspects of the natural environment. At this time, it is difficult to assess these long-term possibilities as the pandemic is still ongoing. In the future, however, it is crucial that research be done in this area.

The formation of this research's framework was an inductive process that required evolution and trial and error. Once an adequate theoretical structure was formed, this framework was applied through two case study examples—one past health crisis and one smaller-scale regional case of the COVID-19 pandemic—in order to assess its transferability and scalability. This process demonstrated that there is ultimately room for improvement and refinement of this framework. More categories can be created or utilized, mechanisms can be added to allow for the framework to account for quantifiable results, and entering and exiting flow pathways can be implemented to account for the movement of impacts in and out of a case on a scaled-down level. But while this theory can be improved, the framework still provides a useful method for approaching a human health crisis with an environmentally-aware mindset. By offering a broad tool with which to assess the environmental impacts of health crises in the future, the goal is that this research can help to bridge the gap in our understanding of the connections between the environment and public health. In the end, many beneficial environmental impacts occurred as a result of the COVID-19 pandemic, but they came at the expense of widespread human suffering and restriction. Over time, many of these benefits were reversed. Ultimately, in moving forward, it is crucial that we develop more sustainable, socially-responsible, and equitable ways to lower our greenhouse gas emissions as a society and reduce our impact on the natural environment.

References

Abu-Qdais, H. A., Al-Ghazo, M. A., & Al-Ghazo, E. M. (2020). Statistical analysis and characteristics of hospital medical waste under novel Coronavirus outbreak. *Global Journal of Environmental Science and Management; Tehran, 6*(4), 1–10. http://dx.doi.org/10.22034/gjesm.2020.04.0

"Addressing Vaccine Waste" (2014). *The UCLA Fielding School of Public Health Magazine.* Retrieved October 25, 2020, from https://ph.ucla.edu/news/magazine/2014/spring/article/addressing-vaccine-waste

Ahmed, W., Angel, N., Edson, J., Bibby, K., Bivins, A., O'Brien, J. W., Choi, P. M., Kitajima, M., Simpson, S. L., Li, J., Tscharke, B., Verhagen, R., Smith, W. J. M., Zaugg, J., Dierens, L., Hugenholtz, P., Thomas, K. V., & Mueller, J. F. (2020). First confirmed detection of SARS-CoV-2 in untreated wastewater in Australia: A proof of concept for the wastewater surveillance of COVID-19 in the community. *Science of The Total Environment, 728*, 138764. https://doi.org/10.1016/j.scitotenv.2020.138764

Ali, F. (2020, August 25). Ecommerce trends amid coronavirus pandemic in charts. *Digital Commerce 360.* https://www.digitalcommerce360.com/2020/08/25/ecommerce-during-coronavirus-pandemic-in-charts/

Allen, R. J., Brenniman, G. R., & Darling, C. (1986). Air Pollution Emissions from the Incineration of Hospital Waste. *Journal of the Air Pollution Control Association, 36*(7), 829–831. https://doi.org/10.1080/00022470.1986.10466122

Arora, S., Bhaukhandi, K. D., & Mishra, P. K. (2020). Coronavirus lockdown helped the environment to bounce back. *The Science of the Total Environment, 742*, 140573. https://doi.org/10.1016/j.scitotenv.2020.140573

Audi, A., AlIbrahim, M., Kaddoura, M., Hijazi, G., Yassine, H. M., & Zaraket, H. (2020). Seasonality of Respiratory Viral Infections: Will COVID-19 Follow Suit? *Frontiers in Public Health, 8.* https://doi.org/10.3389/fpubh.2020.567184

Barnard, A., Paybarah, A., & Meschke, J. (2020, June 2). What New York's Trash Reveals About Life Under Lockdown. *The New York Times.* https://www.nytimes.com/2020/06/02/nyregion/nyc-garbage-pickup-coronavirus.html

Bates, A. E., Primack, R. B., Moraga, P., & Duarte, C. M. (2020). COVID-19 pandemic and associated lockdown as a "global human confinement experiment" to investigate biodiversity conservation. *Biological Conservation, 248*, 108665. https://doi.org/10.1016/j.biocon.2020.108665

Bates, S. (2020, December 4). *AGU Panel Explores Environmental Impacts of the COVID-19 Pandemic.* NASA. http://www.nasa.gov/feature/goddard/2020/agu-panel-explores-environmental-impacts-of-the-covid-19-pandemic-as-observed-from-space

Bauman, A. (2020, July 29). *Trash Piling Up Over NYC After Sanitation Department's Budget Slashed By Over $100 Million.* CBS New York. https://newyork.cbslocal.com/2020/07/29/trash-collection-nyc-sanitation-department-budget-cuts/

Bell, D. M. (2004). Public Health Interventions and SARS Spread, 2003. *Emerging Infectious Diseases, 10*(11), 1900–1906. https://doi.org/10.3201/eid1011.040729

Berliner, U. (2020, July 8). New Yorkers Look To Suburbs And Beyond. Other City Dwellers

May Be Next. *NPR.Org*. Retrieved November 15, 2020, from https://www.npr.org/2020/07/08/887585383/new-yorkers-look-to-suburbs-and-beyond-other-city-dwellers-may-be-next

Berlinger, J. (2020, February 26). Coronavirus has now spread to every continent except Antarctica. *CNN*. Retrieved August 23, 2020, from https://www.cnn.com/2020/02/25/asia/novel-coronavirus-covid-update-us-soldier-intl-hnk/index.html

Bhowmick, G. D., Dhar, D., Nath, D., Ghangrekar, M. M., Banerjee, R., Das, S., & Chatterjee, J. (2020). Coronavirus disease 2019 (COVID-19) outbreak: Some serious consequences with urban and rural water cycle. *Npj Clean Water*, *3*(1), 1–8. https://doi.org/10.1038/s41545-020-0079-1

Borrelli, S. S. (2020, March 9). Italy orders total lockdown over coronavirus. *POLITICO*. https://www.politico.eu/article/italy-orders-total-lockdown-over-coronavirus/

Braga, F., Scarpa, G. M., Brando, V. E., Manfè, G., & Zaggia, L. (2020). COVID-19 lockdown measures reveal human impact on water transparency in the Venice Lagoon. *The Science of the Total Environment*, *736*, 139612. https://doi.org/10.1016/j.scitotenv.2020.139612

Brugger, K. (2020, August 19). *The medical waste crisis that didn't happen—Yet*. E&E News. https://www.eenews.net/stories/1063712043

Brynjolfsson, E., Horton, J. J., Ozimek, A., Rock, D., Sharma, G., & TuYe, H.-Y. (2020). *COVID-19 and Remote Work: An Early Look at US Data* (No. w27344). National Bureau of Economic Research. https://doi.org/10.3386/w27344

Carey, B., & Glanz, J. (2020, April 23). Hidden Outbreaks Spread Through U.S. Cities Far Earlier Than Americans Knew, Estimates Say. The New York Times. https://www.nytimes.com/2020/04/23/us/coronavirus-early-outbreaks-cities.html

Centers for Disease Control and Prevention (2020a). *COVID-19 and Animals*. Centers for Disease Control and Prevention. https://www.cdc.gov/coronavirus/2019-ncov/daily-life-coping/animals.html

Centers for Disease Control and Prevention (2020b). Interim Infection Prevention and Control Recommendations for Healthcare Personnel During the Coronavirus Disease 2019 (COVID-19) Pandemic. *Coronavirus Disease 2019 (COVID-19)*. Centers for Disease Control and Prevention. https://www.cdc.gov/coronavirus/2019-ncov/hcp/infection-control-recommendations.html

Centers for Disease Control and Prevention. (2020c). *Social Distancing*. Centers for Disease Control and Prevention. https://www.cdc.gov/coronavirus/2019-ncov/prevent-getting-sick/social-distancing.html

Centers for Disease Control and Prevention (2020d). Reopening Guidance for Cleaning and Disinfecting Public Spaces, Workplaces, Businesses, Schools, and Homes. *Coronavirus Disease 2019 (COVID-19)*. Centers for Disease Control and Prevention. https://www.cdc.gov/coronavirus/2019-ncov/community/reopen-guidance.html

Centers for Disease Control and Prevention. (2019, April 23). *Quarantine and Isolation*. https://www.cdc.gov/quarantine/index.html

Centers for Disease Control and Prevention (n.d.). *Severe Acute Respiratory Syndrome (SARS) Basics Factsheet*. Retrieved January 10, 2021, from https://www.cdc.gov/sars/about/fs-sars.html

Centers for Disease Control and Prevention (2003). Efficiency of quarantine during an epidemic of severe acute respiratory syndrome--Beijing, China, 2003. MMWR. Morbidity and mortality weekly report, 52(43), 1037–1040. https://pubmed.ncbi.nlm.nih.gov/14586295/

Centre for Research on Energy and Clean Air [CREA]. (2021, May 18). *China's air pollution overshoots pre-crisis levels for the first time.* Centre for Research on Energy and Clean Air [CREA]. https://energyandcleanair.org/

Chan, K. H., Poon, L. L. L. M., Cheng, V. C. C., Guan, Y., Hung, I. F. N., Kong, J., Yam, L. Y. C., Seto, W. H., Yuen, K. Y., & Peiris, J. S. M. (2004). Detection of SARS Coronavirus in Patients with Suspected SARS. Emerging Infectious Diseases, 10(2), 294–299. https://doi.org/10.3201/eid1002.030610

Cheval, S., Teodoro Georgiadis, Herrnegger, M., Piticar, A., Legates, D. R., & Adamescu, Christian Mihai. (2020). Observed and Potential Impacts of the COVID-19 Pandemic on the Environment. *International Journal of Environmental Research and Public Health,* *17*(11). http://dx.doi.org/10.3390/ijerph17114140

Chiang, C. F., Sung, F. C., Chang, F. H., & Tsai, C. T. (2006). Hospital waste generation during an outbreak of severe acute respiratory syndrome in Taiwan. Infection Control and Hospital Epidemiology, 27(5), 519– 522. https://doi.org/10.1086/503691

Chow, A. R. (2020, July 22). *National Parks Are Getting Trashed During COVID-19, Endangering Surrounding Communities.* TIME. Retrieved October 25, 2020, from https://time.com/5869788/national-parks-covid-19/

Chu, C. M., Cheng, V. C. C., Hung, I. F. N., Wong, M. M. L., Chan, K. H., Chan, K. S., Kao, R. Y. T., Poon, L. L. M., Wong, C. L. P., Guan, Y., Peiris, J. S. M., Yuen, K. Y., & HKU/UCH SARS Study Group. (2004). Role of lopinavir/ritonavir in the treatment of SARS: Initial virological and clinical findings. Thorax, 59(3), 252–256. https://doi.org/10.1136/thorax.2003.012658

Chua, J. M. (2020, May 20). *Plastic bags were finally being banned. Then came the pandemic.* Vox. https://www.vox.com/the-goods/2020/5/20/21254630/plastic-bags-single-use-cups-coronavirus-covid-19-delivery-recycling

Convention on Biological Diversity (2010, April 27). What is Impact Assessment? *United Nations Environment Programme.* https://www.cbd.int/impact/whatis.shtml

COVID-19 Mobility Trends Reports. (n.d.). Apple. Retrieved November 15, 2020, from https://www.apple.com/covid19/mobility

Dantas, G., Siciliano, B., França, B. B., da Silva, C. M., & Arbilla, G. (2020). The impact of COVID-19 partial lockdown on the air quality of the city of Rio de Janeiro, Brazil. *Science of The Total Environment, 729,* 139085. https://doi.org/10.1016/j.scitotenv.2020.139085

Dockery, D. W., Pope, C. A., Xu, X., Spengler, J. D., Ware, J. H., Fay, M. E., Ferris, B. G., & Speizer, F. E. (1993). An Association between Air Pollution and Mortality in Six U.S. Cities. *New England Journal of Medicine, 329*(24), 1753–1759. https://doi.org/10.1056/NEJM199312093292401

Documenting New York's path to recovery from the coronavirus (COVID-19) pandemic, 2020-2021. (n.d.). Ballotpedia. Retrieved March 26, 2021, from https://ballotpedia.org/Documenting_New_York%27s_path_to_recovery_from_the_coronavirus_(COVID-19)_pandemic,_2020-2021

Doheny, K. (2020, June 29). *COVID-19 Fallout: Tons of Trash.* WebMD Health News. https://www.webmd.com/lung/news/20200629/covid19-fallout-tons-of-trash

Dunford, D., Dale, B., Stylianou, N., Lowther, E., Ahmed, M., & de la Torre Arenas, I. (2020,

April 7). Coronavirus: The world in lockdown in maps and charts. *BBC News.*
https://www.bbc.com/news/world-52103747

Eckelman, M. J., & Sherman, J. (2016). Environmental impacts of the U.S. health care system and effects on public health. *PLOS ONE, 11*(6), e0157014.
https://doi.org/10.1371/journal.pone.0157014

Environmental and Energy Study Institute [EESI] (2019, October 27). Fact Sheet: The Growth in Greenhouse Gas Emissions from Commercial Aviation.
https://www.eesi.org/papers/view/fact-sheet-the-growth-in- greenhouse-gas-emissions-from-commercial-aviation

European Environment Agency (2020, June 16). Air quality and COVID-19. *European Environment Agency.* Retrieved July 4, 2020, from
https://www.eea.europa.eu/themes/air/air-quality-and-covid19/air-quality-and-covid19

Ewe, K. (2020, May 29). Chinese Authorities Say That the Coronavirus Didn't Originate From the Wuhan Market. *VICE Media Group.* Retrieved October 12, 2020, from
https://www.vice.com/en/article/pkybvv/china-cdc-coronavirus-origin-not-wuhan-market

Fattorini, D., & Regoli, F. (2020). Role of the chronic air pollution levels in the Covid-19 outbreak risk in Italy. *Environmental Pollution (Barking, Essex : 1987), 264,* 114732.
https://doi.org/10.1016/j.envpol.2020.114732

Ferré-Sadurní, L., & Cramer, M. (2020, April 15). New York Orders Residents to Wear Masks in Public. *The New York Times.*
https://www.nytimes.com/2020/04/15/nyregion/coronavirus-face-masks-andrew-cuomo.html

U.S. Food and Drug Administration. (2020a, December 11). FDA Takes Key Action in Fight Against COVID-19 By Issuing Emergency Use Authorization for First COVID-19 Vaccine. Office of the Commissioner, Food and Drug Administration.
https://www.fda.gov/news-events/press-announcements/fda-takes-key-action-fight-against-covid-19-issuing-emergency-use-authorization-first-covid-19

U.S. Food and Drug Administration. (2020b, December 18). FDA Takes Additional Action in Fight Against COVID-19 By Issuing Emergency Use Authorization for Second COVID-19 Vaccine. Office of the Commissioner, Food and Drug Administration.
https://www.fda.gov/news-events/press-announcements/fda-takes-additional-action-fight-against-covid-19-issuing-emergency-use-authorization-second-covid

U.S. Food and Drug Administration. (2021, February 27). *FDA Issues Emergency Use Authorization for Third COVID-19 Vaccine.* FDA; FDA. https://www.fda.gov/news-events/press-announcements/fda-issues-emergency-use-authorization-third-covid-19-vaccine

Florida, R., Glaeser, E., Mohd Sharif, M., Bedi, K., Campanella, T. J., Chee, C. H., Doctoroff, D., Katz, B., Katz, R., Kotkin, J., Muggah, R., & Sadik-Khan, J. (n.d.). How Life in Our Cities Will Look After the Coronavirus Pandemic. *Foreign Policy.* Retrieved November 15, 2020, from https://foreignpolicy.com/2020/05/01/future-of-cities-urban-life-after-coronavirus-pandemic/

Francescani, C. (2020, June 17). *Timeline: The first 100 days of New York Gov. Andrew Cuomo's COVID-19 response.* ABC News. Retrieved February 16, 2021, from
https://abcnews.go.com/US/News/timeline-100-days-york-gov-andrew-cuomos-covid/story?id=71292880

Frost, M., Li, R., Moolenaar, R., Mao, Q., & Xie, R. (2019). Progress in public health risk communication in China: Lessons learned from SARS to H7N9. *BMC Public Health,* *19*(3), 475. https://doi.org/10.1186/s12889-019-6778-1

Gillingham, K. T., Knittel, C. R., Li, J., Ovaere, M., & Reguant, M. (2020). The Short-run and Long-run Effects of Covid-19 on Energy and the Environment. Joule, 4(7), 1337–1341. https://doi.org/10.1016/j.joule.2020.06.010

Goldenberg, S., & Muoio, D. (2020, January 5). *Wasted Potential: The consequences of New York City's recycling failure.* Politico PRO. https://politi.co/39HcdCG

Gorman, J. (2020, February 27). China's Ban on Wildlife Trade a Big Step, but Has Loopholes, Conservationists Say. *The New York Times.* https://www.nytimes.com/2020/02/27/science/coronavirus-pangolin-wildlife-ban-china.html

Griffin, A. (2021, February 3). *DOT to Add 10,000 Bike Parking Racks Throughout City by 2022.* Astoria Post. https://astoriapost.com/dot-to-add-10000-bike-parking-racks-throughout-city-by-2022

Gundy, P. M., Gerba, C. P., & Pepper, I. L. (2008). Survival of Coronaviruses in Water and Wastewater. Food and Environmental Virology, 1(1), 10. https://doi.org/10.1007/s12560-008-9001-6

Gwenzi, W. (2021). Leaving no stone unturned in light of the COVID-19 faecal-oral hypothesis? A water, sanitation and hygiene (WASH) perspective targeting low-income countries. *Science of The Total Environment, 753,* 141751. https://doi.org/10.1016/j.scitotenv.2020.141751

Haag, M., & Rubinstein, D. (2020, December 11). Midtown Is Reeling. Should Its Offices Become Apartments? *The New York Times.* https://www.nytimes.com/2020/12/11/nyregion/nyc-commercial-real-estate.html

Hamwey, R. (2020, April 20). Environmental impacts of coronavirus crisis, challenges ahead. *United Nations Conference on Trade and Development.* Retrieved July 9, 2020, from https://unctad.org/en/pages/newsdetails.aspx?OriginalVersionID=2333

He, E., & Laurent, L. (2020, July 17). The World Is Masking Up, Some Are Opting Out. *Bloomberg.com.* https://www.bloomberg.com/graphics/2020-opinion-coronavirus-global-face-mask-adoption/

He, J.-C., & Xu, Y.-Q. (2012). Estimation of the Aircraft CO_2 Emissions of China's Civil Aviation during 1960–2009. *Advances in Climate Change Research, 3*(2), 99–105. https://doi.org/10.3724/SP.J.1248.2012.00099

Heller, L., Mota, C. R., & Greco, D. B. (2020). COVID-19 faecal-oral transmission: Are we asking the right questions? *Science of The Total Environment, 729,* 138919. https://doi.org/10.1016/j.scitotenv.2020.138919

Helm, D. (2020). The Environmental Impacts of the Coronavirus. *Environmental & Resource Economics,* 1–18. https://doi.org/10.1007/s10640-020-00426-z

Hu, W. (2020, April 9). N.Y.'s Changed Streets: In One Spot, Traffic Speeds Are Up 288%. *The New York Times.* https://www.nytimes.com/2020/04/09/nyregion/nyc-coronavirus-empty-streets.html

Huang, Y. (2004). The SARS Epidemic and its Aftermath in China: A Political Perspective. In Institute of Medicine (2004). *Learning from SARS: Preparing for the Next Disease Outbreak: Workshop Summary.* (pp. 116-132) Washington, DC: The National Academies Press. https://doi.org/10.17226/10915.

Hung, L. S. (2003). The SARS Epidemic in Hong Kong: What Lessons Have We Learned?

Journal of the Royal Society of Medicine, *96*(8), 374–378.
   https://doi.org/10.1177/014107680309600803

Institute of Medicine (2001). *Rebuilding the Unity of Health and the Environment: A New Vision
   of Environmental Health for the 21st Century*. National Academies Press (US).
   http://www.ncbi.nlm.nih.gov/books/NBK99589/

Institute of Medicine (2004). *Learning from SARS: Preparing for the Next Disease Outbreak:
   Workshop Summary*. Washington, DC: The National Academies Press.
   https://doi.org/10.17226/10915.

Institute of Medicine (2013). *Public Health Linkages with Sustainability: Workshop Summary*.
   The National Academies Press. https://www.nap.edu/download/18375

Iwasaki, A. (2020). What reinfections mean for COVID-19. *The Lancet Infectious Diseases*.
   https://doi.org/10.1016/S1473-3099(20)30783-0

Johns Hopkins Center for Systems Science and Engineering (2021). COVID-19 dashboard.
   Johns Hopkins Coronavirus Resource Center, Johns Hopkins University. Retrieved
   March 20, 2021, from https://coronavirus.jhu.edu/map.html

Johns Hopkins Coronavirus Resource Center (2021, January 10). *Mortality Analyses*. Johns
   Hopkins Coronavirus Resource Center. https://coronavirus.jhu.edu/data/mortality

Kerimray, A., Baimatova, N., Ibragimova, O. P., Bukenov, B., Kenessov, B., Plotitsyn, P., &
   Karaca, F. (2020). Assessing air quality changes in large cities during COVID-19
   lockdowns: The impacts of traffic-free urban conditions in Almaty, Kazakhstan. *The
   Science of the Total Environment*, *730*, 139179.
   https://doi.org/10.1016/j.scitotenv.2020.139179

Khafagy, A. (2020, December 23). *With volumes down, New York City commercial waste
   workers struggle to adjust*. Waste Dive. https://www.wastedive.com/news/new-york-
   commercial-waste-workers-pandemic/592580/

Kilgannon, C. (2020, December 8). What New York City's Sewers Reveal About the Virus. *The
   New York Times*. https://www.nytimes.com/2020/12/08/nyregion/covid-testing-
   sewers.html

Klemeš, J. J., Fan, Y. V., Tan, R. R., & Jiang, P. (2020). Minimising the present and future
   plastic waste, energy and environmental footprints related to COVID-19. *Renewable and
   Sustainable Energy Reviews*, *127*, 109883. https://doi.org/10.1016/j.rser.2020.109883

Koh, L. P., Li, Y., & Lee, J. S. H. (2021). The value of China's ban on wildlife trade and
   consumption. *Nature Sustainability*, *4*(1), 2–4. https://doi.org/10.1038/s41893-020-
   00677-0

Kuebelbeck Paulsen, S. (2020, October 26). *Studies show long-term COVID-19 immune
   response*. Center for Infectious Disease Research and Policy, The University of
   Minnesota. https://www.cidrap.umn.edu/news-perspective/2020/10/studies-show-long-
   term-covid-19-immune-response

Kulkarni, B. N., & Anantharama, V. (2020). Repercussions of COVID-19 pandemic on
   municipal solid waste management: Challenges and opportunities. *The Science of the
   Total Environment*, *743*, 140693. https://doi.org/10.1016/j.scitotenv.2020.140693

Landrigan, P., Fuller, R., Acosta, N., Adeyi, O., Arnold, R., Basu, N., Baldé, A., Bertollini, R.,
   Bose-O'Reilly, S., Boufford, J., Breysse, P., Chiles, T., Mahidol, C., Coll-Seck, A.,
   Cropper, M., Fobil, J., Fuster, V., Greenstone, M., Haines, A., & Zhong, M. (2017). The
   Lancet Commission on pollution and health. *The Lancet*, *391*(10119), 462-512.
   https://doi.org/10.1016/S0140-6736(17)32345-0

Lau, J. T. F., Tsui, H., Lau, M., & Yang, X. (2004). SARS Transmission, Risk Factors, and Prevention in Hong Kong. *Emerging Infectious Diseases, 10*(4), 587–592. https://doi.org/10.3201/eid1004.030628

Lee, D. S., Fahey, D. W., Forster, P. M., Newton, P. J., Wit, R. C. N., Lim, L. L., Owen, B., & Sausen, R. (2009). Aviation and global climate change in the 21st century. Atmospheric Environment (Oxford, England : 1994), 43(22), 3520–3537. https://doi.org/10.1016/j.atmosenv.2009.04.024

Le Quéré, C., Jackson, R. B., Jones, M. W., Smith, A. J. P., Abernethy, S., Andrew, R. M., De-Gol, A. J., Willis, D. R., Shan, Y., Canadell, J. G., Friedlingstein, P., Creutzig, F., & Peters, G. P. (2020a). Temporary reduction in daily global CO_2 emissions during the COVID-19 forced confinement. *Nature Climate Change, 10*(7), 647–653. https://doi.org/10.1038/s41558-020-0797-x

Le Quéré, C., Jackson, R., Jones, M., Smith, A., Abernethy, S., Andrew, R., De-Gol, A., Shan, Y., Canadell, J., Friedlingstein, P., Creutzig, F., & Peters, G. (2020b). Supplementary data to: Le Quéré et al (2020), Temporary reduction in daily global CO2 emissions during the COVID-19 forced confinement (Version 1.0). Global Carbon Project. https://doi.org/10.18160/RQDW-BTJU

Liu, W., Tang, F., Fontanet, A., Zhan, L., Zhao, Q.-M., Zhang, P.-H., Wu, X.-M., Zuo, S.-Q., Baril, L., Vabret, A., Xin, Z.-T., Shao, Y.-M., Yang, H., & Cao, W.-C. (2004). Long-term SARS Coronavirus Excretion from Patient Cohort, China. Emerging Infectious Diseases, 10(10), 1841–1843. https://doi.org/10.3201/eid1010.040297

Lokhandwala, S., & Gautam, P. (2020). Indirect impact of COVID-19 on environment: A brief study in Indian context. *Environmental Research, 188*, 109807. https://doi.org/10.1016/j.envres.2020.109807

López-Feldman, A., Chávez, C., Vélez, M. A., Bejarano, H., Chimeli, A. B., Féres, J., Robalino, J., Salcedo, R., & Viteri, C. (2020). Environmental Impacts and Policy Responses to Covid-19: A View from Latin America. *Environmental and Resource Economics.* https://doi.org/10.1007/s10640-020-00460-x

Ma, Y., Lin, X., Wu, A., Huang, Q., Li, X., & Yan, J. (2020). Suggested guidelines for emergency treatment of medical waste during COVID-19: Chinese experience. *Waste Disposal & Sustainable Energy*, 1–4. https://doi.org/10.1007/s42768-020-00039-8

Manzoor, J., & Sharma, M. (2019). Impact of Biomedical Waste on Environment and Human Health. *Environmental Claims Journal, 31*(4), 311–334. https://doi.org/10.1080/10406026.2019.1619265

Martin, D. (1999, May 6). City's Last Waste Incinerator Is Torn Down. *The New York Times.* https://www.nytimes.com/1999/05/06/nyregion/city-s-last-waste-incinerator-is-torn-down.html

Mason, K. A. (2020). Did China's Public Health Reforms Leave It Prepared for COVID-19? *Current History, 119*(818), 203–209. https://doi.org/10.1525/curh.2020.119.818.203

McDonald, L., Simor, A., Su, I.-J., Maloney, S., Ofner, M., Chen, K.-T., Lando, J., Mcgeer, A., Lee, M.-L., & Jernigan, D. (2004). SARS in Healthcare Facilities, Toronto and Taiwan. *Emerging Infectious Diseases, 10*, 777–781. https://doi.org/10.3201/eid1005.030791

Messenger, A. M., Barnes, A. N., & Gray, G. C. (2014). Reverse Zoonotic Disease Transmission (Zooanthroponosis): A Systematic Review of Seldom-Documented Human Biological Threats to Animals. *PLoS ONE, 9*(2). https://doi.org/10.1371/journal.pone.0089055

Metropolitan Transportation Authority. (n.d.). *Day-by-day ridership numbers*. MTA. Retrieved

March 10, 2021, from https://new.mta.info/coronavirus/ridership

Mitjà, O., & Clotet, B. (2020). Use of antiviral drugs to reduce COVID-19 transmission. *The Lancet Global Health, 8*(5), e639–e640. https://doi.org/10.1016/S2214-109X(20)30114-5

Muhammad, S., Long, X., & Salman, M. (2020). COVID-19 pandemic and environmental pollution: A blessing in disguise? *The Science of the Total Environment, 728*, 138820. https://doi.org/10.1016/j.scitotenv.2020.138820

Muoio, D. (2020, July 17). *The coronavirus comeback no one wants: New York City traffic.* Politico. https://politi.co/3eJlKKJ

Nabi, G., & Khan, S. (2020). Risk of COVID-19 pneumonia in aquatic mammals. *Environmental Research, 188*, 109732. https://doi.org/10.1016/j.envres.2020.109732

Nabi, G., Wang, Y., Hao, Y., Khan, S., Wu, Y., & Li, D. (2020). Massive use of disinfectants against COVID-19 poses potential risks to urban wildlife. *Environmental Research, 188*, 109916. https://doi.org/10.1016/j.envres.2020.109916

Nannou, C., Ofrydopoulou, A., Evgenidou, E., Heath, D., Heath, E., & Lambropoulou, D. (2020). Antiviral drugs in aquatic environment and wastewater treatment plants: A review on occurrence, fate, removal and ecotoxicity. *Science of The Total Environment, 699*, 134322. https://doi.org/10.1016/j.scitotenv.2019.134322

National Institute for Public Health and the Environment. (2018, November 12). *Life Cycle Assessment (LCA).* National Institute for Public Health and the Environment; Ministry of Health, Welfare and Sport (Rijksinstituut voor Volksgezondheid en Milieu [RIVM]). https://www.rivm.nl/en/life-cycle-assessment-lca

Needleman, H. L., Gunnoe, C., Leviton, A., Reed, R., Peresie, H., Maher, C., & Barrett, P. (1979). Deficits in psychologic and classroom performance of children with elevated dentine lead levels. *New England Journal of Medicine, 300*(13), 689-695.

New York Forward Phases. (2020, June 8). NYCgo.com. https://www.nycgo.com/coronavirus-information-and-resources-for-travelers/new-york-forward-phases

New York's Next Comeback. (2020, October). Regional Planning Association. https://rpa.org/work/reports/new-yorks-next-comeback

Nir, S. M. (2020, August 27). Trash Piles Up in Parks, Just When New Yorkers Need Them the Most. *The New York Times.* https://www.nytimes.com/2020/08/27/nyregion/nyc-parks-trash.html

New York City Department of Environmental Protection. (n.d.-a). *COVID-19 Wastewater Testing.* Retrieved February 21, 2021, from https://www1.nyc.gov/site/dep/whats-new/covid-19-wastewater-testing.page

New York City Department of Environmental Protection (n.d.-b). *Transportation Emissions.* Retrieved February 23, 2021, from https://www1.nyc.gov/site/dep/environment/transportation-emissions.page

New York City Department of Health and Mental Hygiene. (n.d.-a). *COVID-19: Data Trends.* NYC Health. Retrieved February 16, 2021, from https://www1.nyc.gov/site/doh/covid/covid-19-data-trends.page

New York City Department of Health and Mental Hygiene. (n.d.-b). *COVID-19: Data Totals.* NYC Health. Retrieved February 16, 2021, from https://www1.nyc.gov/site/doh/covid/covid-19-data-totals.page

New York City Department of Health and Mental Hygiene. (n.d.-c). *COVID-19 Vaccination Tracker.* NYC Health. Retrieved February 27, 2021, from https://www1.nyc.gov/site/doh/covid/covid-19-data-vaccines.page

New York City Department of Sanitation. (2020, May 4). *Curbside Composting Updates*. NYC Department of Sanitation (DSNY). Retrieved February 17, 2021, from https://www1.nyc.gov/assets/dsny/site/services/food-scraps-and-yard-waste-page/overview-residents-organics

New York City Department of Sanitation (n.d.-a). *Monthly Reports for DSNY Curbside Collections*. Retrieved March 17, 2021, from https://www1.nyc.gov/assets/dsny/site/resources/statistics/monthly-dsny-curbside-collections

New York City Department of Sanitation. (n.d.-b). *Commercial Waste Zones*. Retrieved April 14, 2021, from https://www1.nyc.gov/assets/dsny/site/resources/reports/commercial-waste-zones-plan

New York State. (2020a, March 20). *Governor Cuomo Signs the "New York State on PAUSE" Executive Order*. Governor Andrew M. Cuomo's Press Office [Press Release]. https://www.governor.ny.gov/news/governor-cuomo-signs-new-york-state-pause-executive-order

New York State. (2020b, September 9). *Governor Cuomo Announces Indoor Dining in New York City Allowed to Resume Beginning September 30 with 25 Percent Occupancy Limit*. Governor Andrew M. Cuomo's Press Office [Press Release]. https://www.governor.ny.gov/news/governor-cuomo-announces-indoor-dining-new-york-city-allowed-resume-beginning-september-30-25

New York State. (2021, March 5). *Governor Cuomo Announces $5 Million in Funding to Support New Pedestrian and Bicycle Path on Manhattan's West Side*. Governor Andrew M. Cuomo's Press Office [Press Release]. https://www.governor.ny.gov/news/governor-cuomo-announces-5-million-funding-support-new-pedestrian-and-bicycle-path-manhattans

New York State. (n.d.-a). *Waste Combustion - Solid Waste Management Facilities Map*. Retrieved February 28, 2021, from https://data.ny.gov/Energy-Environment/Waste-Combustion-Solid-Waste-Management-Facilities/qpvd-9uimc

New York State. (n.d.-b). *Phase One Industries*. New York Forward. Retrieved March 26, 2021, from https://forward.ny.gov/phase-one-industries

New York State. (n.d.-c). *COVID-19 Winter Plan*. New York Forward. Retrieved March 26, 2021, from https://forward.ny.gov/covid-19-winter-plan

New York State. (n.d.-d). *Phased Distribution of the Vaccine*. COVID-19 Vaccine. Retrieved March 26, 2021, from https://covid19vaccine.health.ny.gov/phased-distribution-vaccine

New York State Department of Environmental Conservation. (n.d.). *Regulated Medical Waste*. Retrieved February 23, 2021, from https://www.dec.ny.gov/chemical/8789.html

NYC Mayor's Office of Sustainability (2019). *Inventory of New York City Greenhouse Gas Emissions*. City of New York. https://nyc-ghg-inventory.cusp.nyu.edu/

NYC Open Streets, Open Restaurants to Become Permanent, Year-Round Initiatives. (n.d.). NBC New York. Retrieved February 28, 2021, from https://www.nbcnewyork.com/news/coronavirus/open-streets-and-open-restaurants-to-become-permanent-year-round-initiatives/2636422/

O'Brien, K. (2020, July 9). Ultraviolet lights and HVAC improvements to fight COVID-19. *ABC 8 News*. https://www.wric.com/news/taking-action/ultraviolet-lights-and-hvac-improvements-to-fight-covid-19/

O'Hare, M., & Hardingham-Gill, T. (2020, March 2020). *Coronavirus: Which countries have travel bans?* CNN. Retrieved October 23, 2020, from https://www.cnn.com/travel/article/coronavirus-travel-bans/index.html

Olin, A. (2020, August 5). *Public transit has lost its momentum during the pandemic. Can it be regained?* The Kinder Institute for Urban Research, Rice University. https://kinder.rice.edu/urbanedge/2020/08/05/coronavirus-pandemic-houston-metro-public-transit-ridership

Ouhsine, O., Ouigmane, A., Layati, E., Aba, B., Isaifan, R. J., & Berkani, M. (2020). Impact of COVID-19 on the qualitative and quantitative aspect of household solid waste. *Global Journal of Environmental Science and Management; Tehran, 6*(4), 1–12. http://dx.doi.org/10.22034/gjesm.2020.04.0·

Patino, M. (2020, September 16). What We Actually Know About How Americans Are Moving During Covid. *Bloomberg CityLab.* https://www.bloomberg.com/news/articles/2020-09-16/the-truth-about-american-migration-during-covid

Patz, J. A., Campbell-Lendrum, D., Holloway, T., & Foley, J. A. (2005). Impact of regional climate change on human health. *Nature, 438*(7066), 310–317. https://doi.org/10.1038/nature04188

Paudel, J. (2020). *Short-Run Environmental Effects of COVID-19: Evidence from Forest Fires* (SSRN Scholarly Paper ID 3597247). Social Science Research Network. https://doi.org/10.2139/ssrn.3597247

Pearce, F. (2020, April 7). *After the Coronavirus, Two Sharply Divergent Paths on Climate.* Yale Environment 360, Yale School of the Environment. https://e360.yale.edu/features/after-the-coronavirus-two-sharply-divergent-paths-on-climate

Peevey, A. B., & Cohen, I. (2020, June 12). Residents Fight to Keep Composting From Getting Trashed in New York City's Covid-19 Budget Cuts. *Inside Climate News.* https://insideclimatenews.org/news/12062020/new-york-city-compost-coronavirus/

Peiris, J. S. M., Chu, C. M., Cheng, V. C. C., Chan, K. S., Hung, I. F. N., Poon, L. L. M., Law, K. I., Tang, B. S. F., Hon, T. Y. W., Chan, C. S., Chan, K. H., Ng, J. S. C., Zheng, B. J., Ng, W. L., Lai, R. W. M., Guan, Y., & Yuen, K. Y. (2003). Clinical progression and viral load in a community outbreak of coronavirus-associated SARS pneumonia: A prospective study. *The Lancet, 361*(9371), 1767–1772. https://doi.org/10.1016/S0140-6736(03)13412-5

Perera, F., Berberian, A., Cooley, D., Shenaut, E., Olmstead, H., Ross, Z., & Matte, T. (2021). Potential health benefits of sustained air quality improvements in New York City: A simulation based on air pollution levels during the COVID-19 shutdown. *Environmental Research, 193*, 110555. https://doi.org/10.1016/j.envres.2020.110555

Petersen, E., Koopmans, M., Go, U., Hamer, D. H., Petrosillo, N., Castelli, F., Storgaard, M., Al Khalili, S., & Simonsen, L. (2020). Comparing SARS-CoV-2 with SARS-CoV and influenza pandemics. *The Lancet Infectious Diseases, 20*(9), e238–e244. https://doi.org/10.1016/S1473-3099(20)30484-9

Pham, S. (2020, February 5). SARS cost global airlines $7 billion. The coronavirus outbreak will likely be much worse. CNN. Retrieved January 16, 2021, from https://www.cnn.com/2020/02/05/business/coronavirus-airline-cost/index.html

Plumer, B., & Popovich, N. (2020, June 17). Emissions Are Surging Back as Countries and States Reopen. *The New York Times.* https://www.nytimes.com/interactive/2020/06/17/climate/virus-emissions-reopening.html

Prata, J. C., Silva, A. L. P., Walker, T. R., Duarte, A. C., & Rocha-Santos, T. (2020). COVID-19 Pandemic Repercussions on the Use and Management of Plastics. *Environmental Science & Technology, 54*(13), 7760–7765. https://doi.org/10.1021/acs.est.0c02178

Prüss-Üstün, A., Wolf, J., Corvalán, C., Bos, R., & Neira, M. (2016). *Preventing disease through healthy environments: a global assessment of the burden of disease from environmental risks.* World Health Organization. https://apps.who.int/iris/handle/10665/204585

Race, M., Ferraro, A., Galdiero, E., Guida, M., Núñez-Delgado, A., Pirozzi, F., Siciliano, A., & Fabbricino, M. (2020). Current emerging SARS-CoV-2 pandemic: Potential direct/indirect negative impacts of virus persistence and related therapeutic drugs on the aquatic compartments. *Environmental Research, 188*, 109808. https://doi.org/10.1016/j.envres.2020.109808

Ragazzi, M., Rada, E. C., & Schiavon, M. (2020). Municipal solid waste management during the SARS-COV-2 outbreak and lockdown ease: Lessons from Italy. *The Science of the Total Environment, 745*, 141159. https://doi.org/10.1016/j.scitotenv.2020.141159

Rahman, M. M., Bodrud-Doza, M., Griffiths, M. D., & Mamun, M. A. (2020). Biomedical waste amid COVID-19: Perspectives from Bangladesh. *The Lancet Global Health, 8*(10), e1262. https://doi.org/10.1016/S2214-109X(20)30349-1

Ransom, M. R., & Pope, C. A. (1992). Elementary school absences and PM_{10} pollution in Utah Valley. *Environmental Research, 58*(1), 204–219. https://doi.org/10.1016/S0013-9351(05)80216-6

Redling, A. (2020, March 31). *The first days on the front line.* Waste Today. https://www.wastetodaymagazine.com/article/covid-19-waste-managemnet/

Robinson, B. H. (2009). E-waste: An assessment of global production and environmental impacts. *Science of The Total Environment, 408*(2), 183–191. https://doi.org/10.1016/j.scitotenv.2009.09.044

Salcedo, A., Yar, S., & Cherelus, G. (2020, July 16). Coronavirus travel restrictions, across the globe. *The New York Times.* https://www.nytimes.com/article/coronavirus-travel-restrictions.html

Sanderson, H., Johnson, D. J., Reitsma, T., Brain, R. A., Wilson, C. J., & Solomon, K. R. (2004). Ranking and prioritization of environmental risks of pharmaceuticals in surface waters. *Regulatory Toxicology and Pharmacology, 39*(2), 158–183. https://doi.org/10.1016/j.yrtph.2003.12.006

Satow, J. (2020, August 20). Movers in N.Y.C. Are So Busy They're Turning People Away. *The New York Times.* https://www.nytimes.com/2020/08/20/nyregion/moving-new-york-coronavirus.html

Schaper, D. (2020, October 19). Air Travel High: TSA Screens 1 Million For 1st Time Since March. *NPR.org.* https://www.npr.org/sections/coronavirus-live-updates/2020/10/19/925577175/air-travel-high-tsa-screens-1-million-for-first-time-since-march

Schaye, V. E., Reich, J. A., Bosworth, B. P., Stern, D. T., Volpicelli, F., Shapiro, N., Hauck, K. D., Fagan, I. M., Villagomez, S. M., Uppal, A., Sauthoff, H., LoCurcio, M., Cocks, P. M., & Bails, D. B. (n.d.). Collaborating Across Private, Public, Community, and Federal Hospital Systems: Lessons Learned from the Covid-19 Pandemic Response in NYC. *NEJM Catalyst, 1*(6). https://doi.org/10.1056/CAT.20.0343

Shaw, K. (2006). The 2003 SARS outbreak and its impact on infection control practices. *Public Health, 120*(1), 8–14. https://doi.org/10.1016/j.puhe.2005.10.002

Siciliano, B., Dantas, G., da Silva, C. M., & Arbilla, G. (2020). Increased ozone levels during the COVID-19 lockdown: Analysis for the city of Rio de Janeiro, Brazil. *The Science of the Total Environment, 737*, 139765. https://doi.org/10.1016/j.scitotenv.2020.139765

Silva, P., Prata, J. C., Walker, T. R., Duarte, A. C., Ouyang, W., Barceló, D., & Rocha-Santos, T. (2021). Increased plastic pollution due to COVID-19 pandemic: Challenges and recommendations. *Chemical Engineering Journal, 405*, 126683. https://doi.org/10.1016/j.cej.2020.126683

Singer, A. C. (2018). Antimicrobial use and ecotoxicological risks from pandemics and epidemics. In *Health Care and Environmental Contamination* (pp. 149-165). Elsevier.

Singer, A. C., Colizza, V., Schmitt, H., Andrews, J., Balcan, D., Huang, W. E., ... & Williams, R. J. (2011). Assessing the ecotoxicologic hazards of a pandemic influenza medical

Singh, S., & Prakash, V. (2007). Toxic environmental releases from medical waste incineration: a review. *Environmental Monitoring and Assessment, 132*(1-3), 67-81.

Stawicki, S. P., Jeanmonod, R., Miller, A. C., Paladino, L., Gaieski, D. F., Yaffee, A. Q., De Wulf, A., Grover, J., Papadimos, T. J., Bloem, C., Galwankar, S. C., Chauhan, V., Firstenberg, M. S., Di Somma, S., Jeanmonod, D., Garg, S. M., Tucci, V., Anderson, H. L., Fatimah, L., ... Garg, M. (2020). The 2019–2020 novel coronavirus (Severe Acute Respiratory Syndrome Coronavirus 2) pandemic: A joint American College of Academic International Medicine–World Academic Council of Emergency Medicine multidisciplinary COVID-19 working group consensus paper. *Journal of Global Infectious Diseases, 12*(2), 47–93. https://doi.org/10.4103/jgid.jgid_86_20

Tai, D. Y. H. (2007). Pharmacologic treatment of SARS: Current knowledge and recommendations. Annals of the Academy of Medicine, Singapore, 36(6), 438–443. https://www.annals.edu.sg/pdf/36VolNo6Jun2007/V36N6p438.pdf

The Unexpected Environmental Consequences of COVID-19. (2020, March 30). *Bloomberg Green*. Retrieved July 9, 2020, from https://www.bloomberg.com/news/articles/2020-03-30/the-unexpected-environmental-consequences-of-covid-19

Thompson, C. N., Baumgartner, J., Pichardo, C., Toro, B., Li, L., Arciuolo, R., Chan, P. Y., Chen, J., Culp, G., Davidson, A., Devinney, K., Dorsinville, A., Eddy, M., English, M., Fireteanu, A. M., Graf, L., Geevarughese, A., Greene, S. K., Guerra, K., ... Fine, A. (2020). COVID-19 Outbreak—New York City, February 29–June 1, 2020. *Morbidity and Mortality Weekly Report, 69*(46), 1725–1729. https://doi.org/10.15585/mmwr.mm6946a2

Thomson, B. (2020). The COVID-19 pandemic: A global natural experiment. *Circulation, 142*(1), 14–16. https://doi.org/10.1161/CIRCULATIONAHA.120.047538

Tingley, K. (2020a). Watching What We Flush Could Help Keep a Pandemic Under Control. *The New York Times*. https://www.nytimes.com/2020/11/24/magazine/coronavirus-sewage.html

Tingley, K. (2020b). How Architecture Could Help Us Adapt to the Pandemic. *The New York Times*. https://www.nytimes.com/interactive/2020/06/09/magazine/architecture-covid.html

Tomlinson, B., & Cockram, C. (2003). SARS: Experience at Prince of Wales Hospital, Hong Kong. *The Lancet, 361*(9368), 1486–1487. https://doi.org/10.1016/S0140-6736(03)13218-7

Tsakona, M., Anagnostopoulou, E., & Gidarakos, E. (2006). Hospital waste management and toxicity evaluation: A case study. *Waste Management, 27*(7), 912–920. https://doi.org/10.1016/j.wasman.2006.04.019

Wildlife Conservation Society. (2020, April 22). *Update: Bronx Zoo Tigers and Lions Recovering from COVID-19*. https://newsroom.wcs.org/News-Releases/articleType/ArticleView/articleId/14084/Update-Bronx-Zoo-Tigers-and-Lions-Recovering-from-COVID-19.aspx

United Nations Environment Programme. (2020, August 13). *Waste Management during the COVID-19 Pandemic: From response to recovery*. UN Environment Programme. http://www.unenvironment.org/resources/report/waste-management-during-covid-19-pandemic-response-recovery

U.S. Environmental Protection Agency. (2014, April 9). *Criteria Air Pollutants* [Other Policies and Guidance]. U.S. EPA. https://www.epa.gov/criteria-air-pollutants

U.S. Environmental Protection Agency. (2013, August 31). *What is the National Environmental Policy Act?* [Overviews and Factsheets]. U.S. EPA. https://www.epa.gov/nepa/what-national-environmental-policy-act

United Nations Office on Drugs and Crime (2020, July 10). *UNODC World Wildlife Crime Report 2020: The COVID-19 pandemic has shown that wildlife crime is a threat not only to the environment and biodiversity, but also to human health.* United Nations: Office on Drugs and Crime. Retrieved October 25, 2020, from //www.unodc.org/unodc/en/press/releases/2020/July/unodc-world-wildlife-crime-report-2020_-the-covid-19-pandemic-has-shown-that-wildlife-crime-is-a-threat-not-only-to-the-environment-and-biodiversity--but-also-to-human-health.html

United Nations Department of Economic and Social Affairs (2018, May 16). *68% of the world population projected to live in urban areas by 2050, says UN*. https://www.un.org/development/desa/en/news/population/2018-revision-of-world-urbanization-prospects.html

Varlik, N. (2020, October 14). *How do pandemics end? History suggests diseases fade but are almost never truly gone*. The Conversation. Retrieved November 1, 2020, from http://theconversation.com/how-do-pandemics-end-history-suggests-diseases-fade-but-are-almost-never-truly-gone-146066

Walker, B. L., & Cooper, C. D. (1992). Air Pollution Emission Factors for Medical Waste Incinerators. *Journal of the Air & Waste Management Association, 42*(6), 784–791. https://doi.org/10.1080/10473289.1992.10467030

Wallace, G. (2020, April 9). *Airlines and TSA report 96% drop in air travel*. CNN. https://www.cnn.com/2020/04/09/politics/airline-passengers-decline/index.html

Wang, X.-W., Li, J.-S., Guo, T.-K., Zhen, B., Kong, Q.-X., Yi, B., Li, Z., Song, N., Jin, M., Xiao, W.-J., Zhu, X.-M., Gu, C.-Q., Yin, J., Wei, W., Yao, W., Liu, C., Li, J.-F., Ou, G.-R., Wang, M.-N., … Li, J.-W. (2005). Concentration and detection of SARS coronavirus in sewage from Xiao Tang Shan Hospital and the 309th Hospital. *Journal of Virological Methods, 128*(1), 156–161. https://doi.org/10.1016/j.jviromet.2005.03.022

Wang, Q., & Su, M. (2020). A preliminary assessment of the impact of COVID-19 on environment—A case study of China. *The Science of the Total Environment, 728*, 138915. https://doi.org/10.1016/j.scitotenv.2020.138915

WGRZ Staff. (2020, October 19). *DEC enforcement of New York's plastic bag ban to begin October 19*. wgrz.com. https://www.wgrz.com/article/news/local/dec-enforcement-of-new-yorks-plastic-bag-ban-to-take-place-october-19/71-e6055082-e0fd-4021-8840-2f753247f2a3

Wilder-Smith, A. (2006). The severe acute respiratory syndrome: Impact on travel and tourism.

Travel Medicine and Infectious Disease, 4(2), 53–60.
https://doi.org/10.1016/j.tmaid.2005.04.004

Winters, J. (2020, June 11). Great, now the ocean is filled with COVID trash: Masks, gloves, and hand sanitizer. *Grist*. https://grist.org/climate/great-now-the-ocean-is-filled-with-covid-trash-masks-gloves-and-hand-sanitizer/

World Health Organization (2020a). *Shortage of personal protective equipment endangering health workers worldwide*. Retrieved October 12, 2020, from https://www.who.int/news-room/detail/03-03-2020-shortage-of-personal-protective-equipment-endangering-health-workers-worldwide

World Health Organization (2020b). WHO Director-General's opening remarks at the media briefing on COVID-19 – 11 March 2020. Retrieved August 23, 2020, from https://www.who.int/dg/speeches/detail/who-director-general-s-opening-remarks-at-the-media-briefing-on-covid-19---11-march-2020

World Health Organization. (2003a, March 12). *WHO issues a global alert about cases of atypical pneumonia*. Retrieved January 21, 2021, from https://www.who.int/csr/sars/archive/2003_03_12/en/

World Health Organization. (2003b, March 15). *World Health Organization issues emergency travel advisory*. Retrieved January 21, 2021, from https://www.who.int/csr/sars/archive/2003_03_15/en/

World Health Organization. (2003c, April 23). *WHO extends its SARS-related travel advice to Beijing and Shanxi province in China and to Toronto, Canada*. Retrieved January 21, 2021, from https://www.who.int/mediacentre/news/notes/2003/np7/en/

World Health Organization (n.d.). *Severe Acute Respiratory Syndrome (SARS)*. Retrieved January 10, 2021, from https://www.who.int/health-topics/severe-acute-respiratory-syndrome#tab=tab_1

Yang, Y., Peng, F., Wang, R., Guan, K., Jiang, T., Xu, G., Sun, J., & Chang, C. (2020). The deadly coronaviruses: The 2003 SARS pandemic and the 2020 novel coronavirus epidemic in China. *Journal of Autoimmunity*, *109*, 102434. https://doi.org/10.1016/j.jaut.2020.102434

Yuan, J., & Morgan, R. (2020, March 24). The New York City subway empties—And part of the carnival of life vanishes. *Washington Post*. Retrieved February 18, 2021, from https://www.washingtonpost.com/national/the-new-york-city-subway-empties--and-part-of-the-carnival-of-life-vanishes/2020/03/24/05d69ad4-6df1-11ea-a3ec-70d7479d83f0_story.html

Zambrano-Monserrate, M. A., Ruano, M. A., & Sanchez-Alcalde, L. (2020). Indirect effects of COVID-19 on the environment. *The Science of the Total Environment*, *728*, 138813. https://doi.org/10.1016/j.scitotenv.2020.138813

Zangari, S., Hill, D. T., Charette, A. T., & Mirowsky, J. E. (2020). Air quality changes in New York City during the COVID-19 pandemic. *The Science of the Total Environment*, *742*, 140496. https://doi.org/10.1016/j.scitotenv.2020.140496

Zhang, H., Tang, W., Chen, Y., & Yin, W. (2020). Disinfection threatens aquatic ecosystems. *Science*, *368*(6487), 146–147. https://doi.org/10.1126/science.abb8905

Zhao, L., Zhang, F.-S., Wang, K., & Zhu, J. (2009). Chemical properties of heavy metals in typical hospital waste incinerator ashes in China. Waste Management, 29(3), 1114–1121. https://doi.org/10.1016/j.wasman.2008.09.003

Zhou, P., Yang, X.-L., Wang, X.-G., Hu, B., Zhang, L., Zhang, W., Si, H.-R., Zhu, Y., Li, B.,

Huang, C.-L., Chen, H.-D., Chen, J., Luo, Y., Guo, H., Jiang, R.-D., Liu, M.-Q., Chen, Y., Shen, X.-R., Wang, X., ... Shi, Z.-L. (2020). A pneumonia outbreak associated with a new coronavirus of probable bat origin. *Nature, 579*(7798), 270–273. https://doi.org/10.1038/s41586-020-2012-7

Zhu, N., Zhang, D., Wang, W., Li, X., Yang, B., Song, J., Zhao, X., Huang, B., Shi, W., Lu, R., Niu, P., Zhan, F., Ma, X., Wang, D., Xu, W., Wu, G., Gao, G. F., Tan, W., & China Novel Coronavirus Investigating and Research Team (2020). A novel coronavirus from patients with pneumonia in China, 2019. *The New England Journal of Medicine, 382*(8), 727–733. https://doi.org/10.1056/NEJMoa2001017

Appendix A

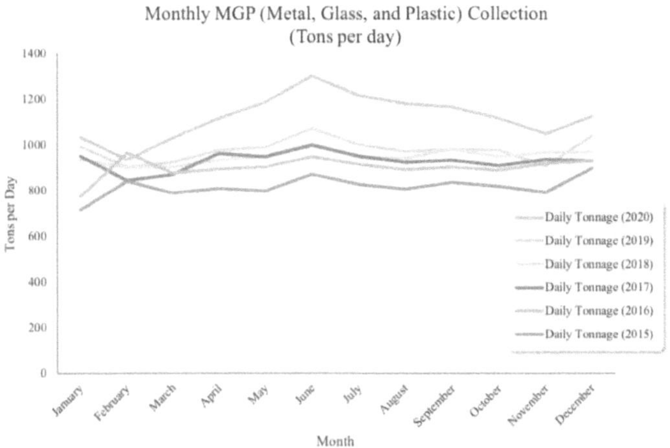

Figure A-1. Monthly residential MGP collection in New York City for the years of 2015 to 2019.

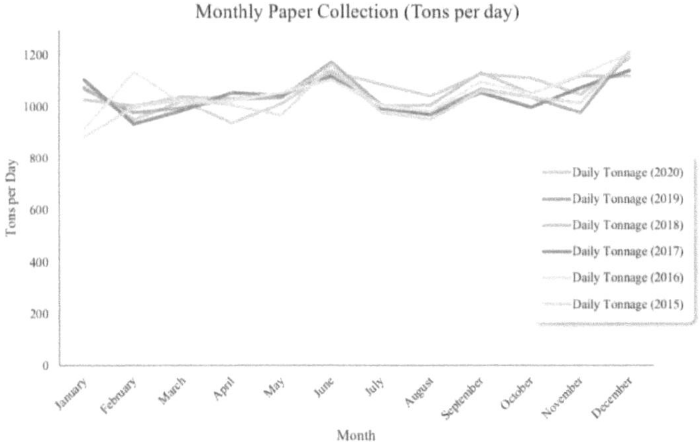

Figure A-2. Monthly residential paper collection in New York City for the years of 2015 to 2019.

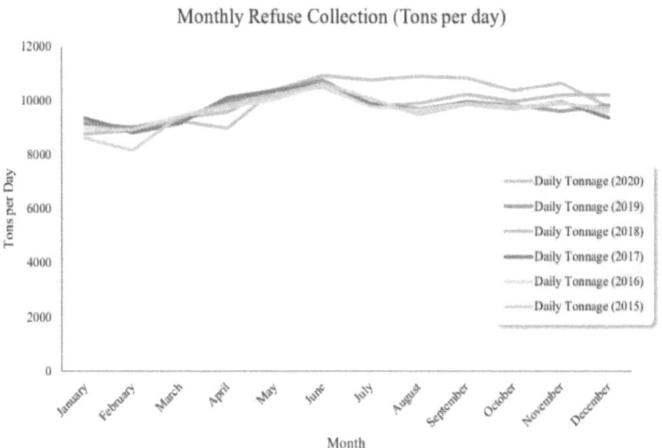

Figure A-3. Monthly residential refuse collection in New York City for the years of 2015 to 2019.

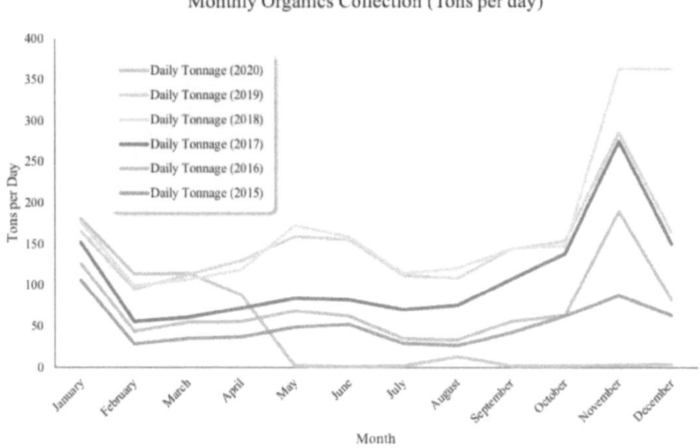

Figure A-4. Monthly residential organics collection in New York City for the years of 2015 to 2019.

116

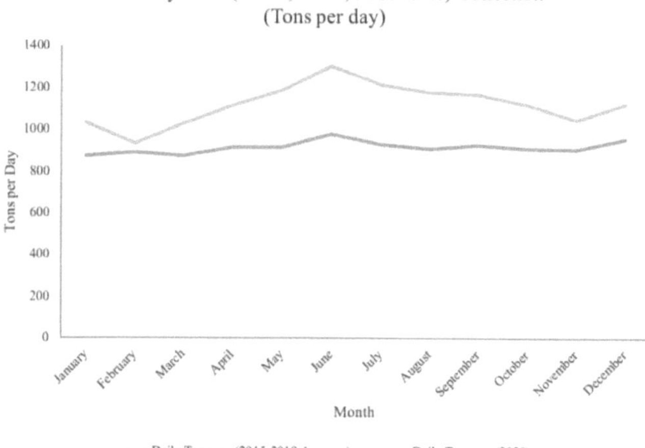

Figure A-5. 2020 monthly residential MGP collection comparison to 2015-2019 calculated monthly average in New York City.

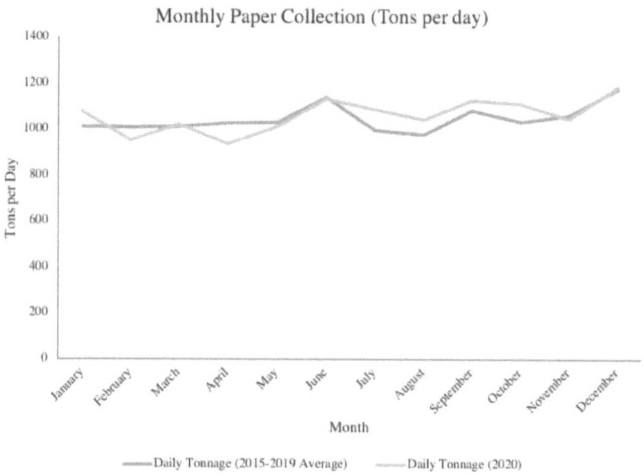

Figure A-6. 2020 monthly residential paper collection comparison to 2015-2019 calculated monthly average in New York City.

117

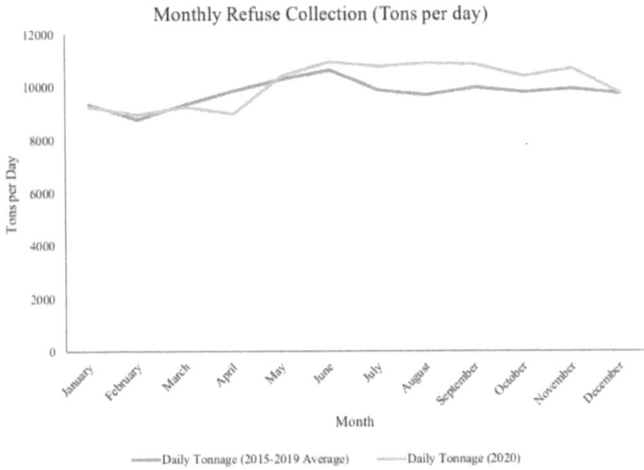

Figure A-7. 2020 monthly residential refuse collection comparison to 2015-2019 calculated monthly average in New York City.

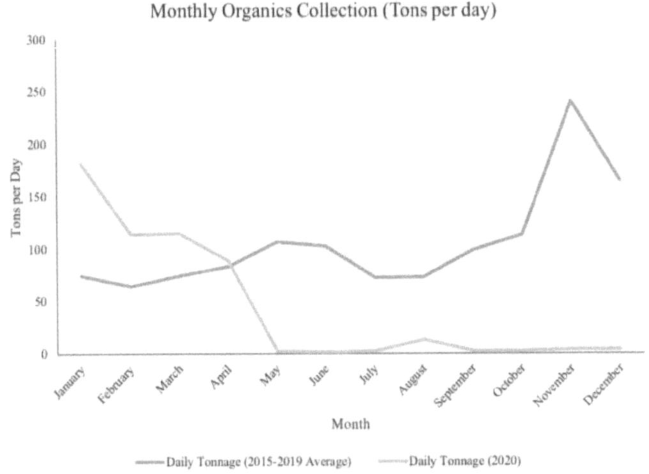

Figure A-8. 2020 monthly residential organics collection comparison to 2015-2019 calculated monthly average in New York City.